Sure, you know how to "v   d,
girl. Now put that positive
Slim Down Sister arr

- The critical role Afri   ..auiuons and
culture play in contributing to obesity

- Easy-to-fix soul-food recipes that keep the
flava but lose the fat

- Tips, strategies, and words of wisdom for staying
focused, motivated, and committed

- The Sister Circle—how to start your own
support group

Slim Down Sister will show you how to keep the weight off
without sacrificing the foods you love. You'll discover the
pleasures of eating right and taking care of your body,
and enjoy the benefits of improved health and a
rejuvenated spirit.

Roniece Weaver and **Fabiola Gaines** are cofounders of Hebni Nutrition Consultants, Inc., a nonprofit organization committed to improving consumers' health by providing comprehensive nutritional information. Weaver is a member of the American Dietetic Association (ADA) and has been a guest speaker for the American Heart Association. Gaines is coordinator of the Women, Infant and Children (WIC) Supplemental Food Program for Florida's Department of Health, and a member of the ADA.
Angela Ebron is a senior editor and writer at *Family Circle* magazine and has contributed to *Essence* and *Child* magazines.

SLIM DOWN SISTER

❖

THE AFRICAN-AMERICAN WOMAN'S GUIDE TO HEALTHY, PERMANENT WEIGHT LOSS

❖

Roniece Weaver, M.S., R.D., L.D.,
Fabiola Gaines, R.D., L.D.,
and Angela Ebron

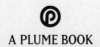

A PLUME BOOK

A NOTE TO THE READER: The ideas, procedures, and suggestions contained in this book are not intended as a substitute for consulting with your physician. All matters regarding your health require medical supervision.

PLUME
Published by the Penguin Group
Penguin Putnam Inc., 375 Hudson Street, New York, New York 10014, U.S.A.
Penguin Books Ltd, 27 Wrights Lane, London W8 5TZ, England
Penguin Books Australia Ltd, Ringwood, Victoria, Australia
Penguin Books Canada Ltd, 10 Alcorn Avenue, Toronto, Ontario, Canada M4V 3B2
Penguin Books (N.Z.) Ltd, 182–190 Wairau Road, Auckland 10, New Zealand

Penguin Books Ltd, Registered Offices: Harmondsworth, Middlesex, England

Published by Plume, a member of Penguin Putnam Inc.
Previously published in a Dutton edition.

First Plume Printing, January 2001
10 9 8 7 6 5 4 3 2 1

Ⓟ REGISTERED TRADEMARK—MARCA REGISTRADA

The Library of Congress has catalogued the Dutton edition as follows:
Weaver, Roniece.
Slim down sister : the African-American woman's guide to healthy, permanent
weight loss / by Roniece Weaver, Fabiola D. Gaines, and Angela Ebron.
        p. cm.
ISBN 0-525-94458-3 (hc.)
   0-452-28060-5 (pbk.)
1. Weight loss. 2. Afro-American women—Health and hygiene.
I. Gaines, Fabiola. II. Ebron, Angela. III. Title.
RM222.2.W2956 2000
613.2'5'08996073—dc21   99-16262

Printed in the United States of America
Original hardcover design by Leonard Telesca

To my mother, Ernestine Williams, and my mother-in-law, Zelma Weaver, and to the memory of my dad—R.W.

To my daughter, Devona, and in memory of my parents, John L. Demps Sr. and Bernetha Sirmans Demps—F.G.

In memory of my grandmothers, Millie Jane Galloway and Gertrude Ebron—A.E.

Contents

SLIM DOWN SISTER

Introduction

You know the feeling. You hit the bookstores, searching for the right guide to help you shed pounds and get in shape. But every weight-loss book you pick up seems to be speaking to some other woman. The diets tout bland, boring, no-soul food. The fitness routines require all sorts of costly gadgets and gear. And the advice . . . well, let's just say a sister was definitely not consulted. That's why we need our own weight loss program. Something tailored specifically to African-American women's concerns.

The fact is, black women are getting heavier. Fifty-two percent of us are obese, according to the Third National Health and Nutrition Examination Study (NHANES III) conducted by the Centers for Disease Control. And the numbers show no sign of slowing down. When you consider that there are 17.8 million black women in the United States, the implication is frightening. Approximately 9 million of us are risking our lives every day because of our weight, no matter how well we may carry it. Make no mistake, obesity can kill. Research shows that life-threatening diseases like hypertension, diabetes, heart disease, and certain forms of cancer can all be directly linked to severe overweight—

and thousands of us are dying of these illnesses every year. According to the National Center for Health Statistics, 31 percent of black women suffer from high blood pressure. In 1993, 23 percent of the deaths of African-American women were attributed to high blood pressure, compared to 5 percent of white women (the most recent figures available from the NHANES III). The same study also shows that diabetes claimed the lives of 27 percent of African-American women, nearly three times the number of white women killed by the same disease.

Keep in mind that you don't have to be severely overweight to suffer weight-related health problems. With each additional pound you put more pressure on your heart and lungs. Digestive diseases, reproductive problems, and obstetrical complications can also be tied to creeping weight. Because black women are twice as likely as white women to be heavy, shedding those excess pounds is a much more pressing issue for us.

So why aren't sisters as fit as their white counterparts? Biology is one factor. A 1996 study by researchers at the University of Pennsylvania found that African-American women have slower metabolisms, burning nearly one hundred fewer calories at rest per day than white women.

The main reason, however, is cultural. Black women simply view issues of weight differently from the way white women do. From our positive self-image and affinity for soul food, to our need for rest and rejuvenation, who we are as black folks has more to do with our difficulty losing weight than we realize.

Chances are, when we look in the mirror we like what we see. Several studies, including research by Shiriki Kumanyika, Ph.D., professor of nutrition and epidemiology at the University of Illinois in Chicago, confirm that we don't view a little "meat on our bones" as a bad thing, but white women do. In her 1993 study, Dr. Kumanyika discovered that approximately 40 percent of moderately and severely overweight black women considered their bodies "attractive" or "very attractive," indicating a positive body image. As much as this high self-esteem is a good thing, it is in many ways, a drawback that can compromise our future health. We may be conscious of our weight—thinking somewhere in the back of our minds that we could stand to drop a few pounds. But as long as we've "got it going on," and the folks in our community don't see excess weight as a negative, we really don't feel much pressure to start or stick with a get-fit plan.

Our views on food also set us apart from white women. What self-respecting sister would ever cook collards without ham hock seasoning? Or serve dinner without homemade cornbread? Many of our food preferences are steeped in Southern tradition, and soul food is a part of our cultural identity. Unfortunately, the high-protein, high-fat, high-sodium, high-sugar content of our menus work against us, packing on the pounds and contributing to our alarmingly high levels of hypertension and diabetes.

White women, on the other hand, are more apt to place health concerns first when it comes to food, selecting low-fat, low-calorie dishes. The bottom line is that we simply aren't as preoccupied with dieting as white women. If we do decide to "cut back," we don't want to give up favorite foods prepared the way we like them.

We also don't want to give up relaxation. According to a recent Pennsylvania State College of Medicine study, African-Americans consider rest more important than exercise. Those surveyed reported that working out adds more stress to their already stressful lives. They'd much rather kick back and relax than hit the gym. Several other studies also show that black folks spend less leisure time exercising than do white Americans. The weekend finds us taking it easy, not in-line skating or jogging. We also shy away from exercise because of the scarcity of affordable and accessible fitness programs in the black community.

Think black women don't need a special fitness routine? Consider this: We have a higher ratio of fat to lean body mass than Caucasian women, and we tend to carry our excess weight in the waist-to-hip area. Don't forget about our slower metabolism. An everywoman exercise program that doesn't take these specifics into account wouldn't do much of anything for us.

The Solution for Sisters

Girlfriend, all of your bookstore searching has finally paid off. We know what doesn't work for you, and more important, we know why. Those other diet books aren't homing in on your specific needs. *Slim Down Sister* does. Whether you want to lose 10 pounds, 25, 50, 100, or more, this book can help. Why? Because we offer you insight into why weight loss is more difficult for African-American women, and we pull no punches. We're honest about the facets of our lifestyle that keep us from our weight-loss goals. We'll key you in to the special health risks associated with overweight that black women face, and help you understand how resolving to get fit is the first step to prolonging your life. We'll show you how to take the best parts of sisterhood—like our positive self-image—and make them work for you, not against you.

Worried about giving up all those tasty foods? Don't be. Within these pages you'll find a Soul Food Pyramid (pages 86–87), chock-full of nutritionally sound food choices that satisfy our particular preferences. We also provide you with a daily food plan—devised with black women in mind—to help you trim down. Best of all, *Slim Down Sister* shows you how to make favorite soul food and Caribbean-influenced dishes more healthful without sacrificing any of that good flavor.

This book will help you work that body, too. Sister-trainer Mara Hoskin-Thomas, a certified fitness professional who has trained hundreds of black women of all shapes and sizes, has created an exercise program designed especially for us. It's a combo routine: easy-to-do aerobics, body resistance exercises, and weight-training moves. No matter how much you might hate working out, Mara's going to get you moving. Your heart will be pumping, your muscles will be working. Girl, you're gonna sweat—and you're going to have a good time doing it. Don't believe us? Then keep reading and you'll discover how to make exercise fun. What's more, this workout won't make unreasonable demands on your time. Mara's effective, any-time workout is easy to fit into your daily routine, no matter how much you've got going on. Because her program is divided into three different weight-loss categories, you'll be able to work out in the manner most appropriate for your body. As Mara explains, heavier people need to be introduced to a fitness program more slowly and gradually. Depending on your level of physical fitness, we'll start you off with a simple yet effective walking program and some body resistance moves, followed by increased aerobic activity and weight training.

You don't have to buy a $1,000 health club membership or spend hours working out to shape up. You can sculpt a new physique in your own home—without spending a ton of money, using special equipment, or making it an all-day affair. All it takes is this exercise program designed specifically for sisters.

Need a support network? We empower you to create your own by showing you how to organize a church-based weight-loss program at your house of worship. You'll find additional moral support in every chapter. Inspirational success stories from sister-friends just like you will help you stay motivated and committed.

Handling plateaus, stumbling blocks, saboteurs, staying on track, and maintaining your success—it's all within these pages. Just think: With one turn of the page you'll improve your health and prolong your life. So go ahead—slim down, sister.

CHAPTER 1

✻

A New Attitude

Do you have control of your life? Many black women would automatically say "Yes." Their finances are in order, they're doing well on the job, their marriages are solid and their kids are healthy, or they're happily single. Things are moving along just fine. They've really "got it together."

Well, we're not talking about your finances, your job, or your relationships. We're talking about your life—literally. Think about it this way: Being in control of your life means having the power to ensure that you live as well as possible. Not materially, but physically. So are you in control?

If you weigh more than is healthy, the answer is no. Why? Because the health risks associated with excess weight, namely heart disease, hypertension, diabetes, and certain cancers, can kill you. And a sister who truly has control of her life would never put herself in that position.

It's easy to understand why so many of us are lax about something so serious. Weight isn't a big issue in the black community. We don't view excess pounds as negatively as white folks do, perhaps because we see it all around us. Far too many of us are overweight. When you see yourself reflected in this many other women every day, what you see becomes the norm. It doesn't bother you or surprise you. You accept it.

Folks in our communities are less apt to belittle a full-figured sister, especially if she knows how to hook up her look. Even though we're bombarded with media images of waif-thin models and actresses, when we go home it's a whole different world. Yes, we have super-skinny sisters in our neighborhoods, too. But many of the rest of us are heavy. Think about your own family. How many of your female relatives are full-figured? It's no wonder we tend to put less emphasis on size than white women do.

Some experts have criticized the standard method for determining fatness—by body mass measurement—as flawed because it doesn't take African-Americans' larger frames and heavier bones into account. But we can simply look around us to see that overweight is a very real problem, especially for black women. Whether obese, moderately overweight, or merely 20 pounds too heavy, the point is that those extra pounds snatch the reins of control right out of your hands.

Girl, You Look Good

Another reason we take less of a hard view of overweight is our strong sense of self. Sisters are known for it. We have no problem patting ourselves on the back. You know the saying: You better blow your own horn because no one else is going to do it for you. Well, black women take that motto to heart. Perhaps it stems from our matriarchal background, or maybe it's due to the societal battles we face today. Whatever the catalyst, black women have developed a deeply rooted self-esteem that shapes our ideas about beauty.

In the black community, weight is no match for style because we don't adhere to the same "ideal" images as whites. As Maya Angelou reminds us, "the span of my hips ... the swing in my waist ... the ride of my breasts" are to be appreciated. And we do. We walk with a purposeful stride, a smile on our lips. We know we look good. Brothers know it too. If you're "working it," you're bound to hear a few appreciative remarks, no matter your size. To us, attractive and overweight aren't mutually exclusive. For many white women, however, excess weight is intolerable. A 1992 study, published in the *International Journal of Eating Disorders*, that compared body images and body-size perceptions among black and white women found that white women were more dissatisfied with their figures and more inclined to view excess weight as a negative. A University of South Carolina study yielded similar results: African-American women indicated less of a desire to be a smaller size than did Caucasian women. It seems black women are much more at ease with their figures, whether size 10, 16, or 22.

Our love of self starts early. Black teenage girls are happier with their bodies than white girls of the same age, according to research at the University of Arizona College of Medicine. Seventy percent of African-American girls reported satisfaction with their current weight, while a whopping 90 percent of Caucasian girls viewed their bodies negatively. What's interesting is that black girls are typically heavier than white girls, according to a study from the National Heart, Lung and Blood Institute.

So what does all of this say about sisters? Does it mean we just don't care how fat we are? Not at all. It simply means we don't beat ourselves up for being full-figured. We focus on the positive, hooking up our outfits to flaunt our curves, not hide them.

Of course, we know when we've reached our weight threshold. The problem is, we tend to base it on aesthetics rather than health. As long as we can dress well, feel confident about our appearance when we step out the door, and elicit a positive reaction from others, we're good to go. It's only when those things falter that we start to worry.

So you say to yourself, "I've got to do something about my weight," and resolve to start a diet. But you know what? That approach to weight loss is bound to fail because you're doing it for the wrong reason. What's to keep you committed when you shed a few pounds and are able to fit back into those outfits? Not a thing. Oh, you'll look good because you're a sister who knows how to "work it," and you carry your weight well. But when those pounds start creeping on again—and they will—you're back to square one. It's a vicious cycle that can only be stopped one way. A new attitude.

It's not about looking good, it's about *feeling* good. Remember, you're taking control of you life.

A Change for the Better

Changing a lifelong way of thinking won't be easy. But it is possible. The first step is to take personal inventory and be honest with yourself. Really think about how well you feel from day to day. Are you often tired? Does mild exertion—say, climbing a flight of stairs—leave you winded? How well do you sleep? Do you ever feel pain in your joints? Do you have any respiratory problems? How's your blood pressure?

By shifting the focus away from your appearance and onto your well-being, you'll start to see the true relationship between weight and health. Once you make that connection, you'll be in a better position to slim down for good.

True weight-loss success comes when you resolve to make an investment in your health. Concentrate on the years you'll add to your life. Then think about the quality of those years. Wouldn't you rather lead a high-quality life that's full of energy and stamina, that's not plagued by illness and disease?

You're nodding your head, but a part of you is afraid you'll have to make drastic changes in order to get there—changes you're not sure you can sustain. Adopting a healthy way of thinking doesn't mean adopting a stringent, food-phobic attitude. You only have to look at white American culture to see where that leads. White women are more prone than sisters to eating disorders, such as bulimia and anorexia, because many of them slip into a body dysmorphia trap. Their body image becomes so distorted that they binge and purge, or avoid food altogether.

Don't be fooled, though. Black women aren't immune to eating disorders. If we continue to focus on the aesthetic issues surrounding weight rather than the health issues, we run the risk of developing a distorted body image as well. We'll simply move from one extreme to the other. That's why it's so crucial for sisters to let go of the "How do I look?" mentality and get with a "How do I feel?" frame of mind.

The goal isn't to lose weight at any cost, by any means. The goal is to develop a healthy relationship with food while improving the poor nutrition and exercise habits that cause far too many of us to become overweight.

It's Time to Get Real

Let's face it. No matter how fine a woman is, if she's overweight, society holds her in lower regard. Why else would an organization like the National Association to Advance Fat Acceptance exist? Fatness is the last bastion for out-and-out discrimination. Yet many sisters simply don't recognize it. In her 1993 study of weight-related attitudes and behaviors of black women, Shiriki Kumanyika, Ph.D., of the University of Illinois, asked obese sisters if being overweight had ever caused them difficulty in getting a job. Almost every single one of them (an astounding 96 percent) said "not to my knowledge," although the reality is probably very different.

The hard truth is that fatness can be a drawback, and not just in the workplace. Take a look at any magazine, movie, television show, or music video. Odds are, the beautiful woman peering back at you, like Halle, Whitney, or Vanessa, wears a size 6, not a 16. Thin is definitely in.

Even our most famous and beautiful sisters aren't immune to the power of judgment. Take Janet Jackson. Her whole demeanor changed once she toned up. Do you remember her ever showing so much skin when she was plump? Even Oprah, who's waged a public battle of the bulge for years, seems to emit a stronger sense of self now that she's slimmed down. Sisters like Janet and Oprah, who live their lives in the public eye, can't help but understand the standard by which we are all judged. Right or wrong, thin and average-weight people, men and women alike, view overweight people differently. They're seen as having no self-control, no willpower.

For heavy sisters, weight prejudice may be overshadowed by the harsher sting of race and gender discrimination. We *know* when that happens. There's no doubt in our minds. Because weight is less of an issue in our community, it doesn't always spring to mind as a cause when we lose ground. We rarely think, "Hmmm. I wonder if I didn't get that job because of my size."

What black women need to realize is that the size of our bodies is as much a factor in how we're viewed and treated as our sex or race. That said, why not resolve to take the weight factor out of the equation?

Take Care of You: Body, Mind, and Soul

We know you have a lot going on: work, family, friends. You lead a demanding life that leaves precious little time for self. When you do have a few moments alone—your own time—you probably want to do a bit of inner work. Soothing your spirit, calming your mind. You deserve that TLC. Your body craves it. What you may not realize is that pampering encompasses far more than a long soak in a hot bath, or 15 minutes of quiet meditation.

The true definition of "pamper" is "to treat with extreme care and attention." What better way to take care of yourself than with good, high-quality foods and enjoyable physical activity. Being healthy is the best kind of pampering possible. Think about how good you'll feel after a tasty, nutritious meal that leaves you satisfied and energetic, rather than bloated and sluggish. Working up a sweat is a great rejuvenator as well. Exercise releases feel-good brain chemicals, like endorphins, which give you a sense of well-being. See how it all adds up?

No one expects you to change your lifestyle overnight. And make no mistake, that's what committing to get fit is: a lifestyle change. Once you take that first step, it's not going to be for a few weeks or a few months. No girlfriend, when you truly resolve to better your health, it's for the rest of your life. Adopting healthier eating habits and adhering to a fitness program is an ongoing process that becomes easier and easier, especially once you begin to feel the benefits: more energy, better stamina, less illness, greater strength. The pounds will dissolve too, but trust us, you'll be feeling so well that sleekness becomes secondary. Experts say it takes twenty-one days to form a habit. Pass that three-week mark and you're well on your way. So get on it, girl. It's time to take control—of your way of thinking, of your weight, of your health. It's time to take control of your life.

Sister to Sister
XOXOXOXOX

Dorothy Robinson, a forty-two-year-old education training specialist from Waterford, Michigan
Current weight: 145 pounds
Amount lost: 15 pounds

About five years ago I was at my heaviest, 160 pounds. I felt sluggish. I didn't have a lot of energy. The thing is, I used to be very active, but at that time I was doing a lot of traveling and eating out—eating just about everything—and I wasn't exercising on a regular basis. Then I got sick. I think it came from being run-down. That's when I really started putting on the pounds.

When you're younger, you might put on a few pounds and think, "Oh, I can get this off." But as you get older, especially if you're not engaged in some kind of physical activity, it's easier to put the weight on and much harder to take it off.

Even though I realized it would be more difficult to lose the weight I was gaining, I didn't do anything about it until I had a reality check. I'd always worn my clothes a bit loose, but during this time five years ago, I noticed that they were getting a little tighter and tighter. You know what I told myself? "I'm going to have to buy more expensive clothes because these are shrinking." Can you believe it? Anyway, back to my reality check. I'd gone to visit family for the holidays and my nine-year-old cousin said, "Something's different about Dot. She's fat!" That's when it dawned on me that my clothes weren't getting smaller, I was getting bigger.

That night I went home and threw out all my junk food—especially my two favorites, potato chips and cookies. I decided to start baking my meats and stocking up on vegetables and fruit. I really concentrated on creating dishes that were healthy, and I set up a little routine for myself: When I went to the market on the weekend I'd load up on all the fruit, vegetables, lean meats, and other ingredients I needed, then I'd prepare prepackaged meals. For instance, I made homemade soups and froze them. That way everything was done and I didn't have to make so much of an effort later on. I figured it was the best way for me to develop good eating habits.

In the past, when I'd put on weight, I'd drink a Slim Fast or one of those protein drinks. I'd have two of those and one meal each day. Yeah, I lost weight, but it would never stay off. As soon as I put food in my mouth, I'd gain even more.

I'll tell you about another reality check that opened my eyes to what I needed to do. I used to be a runner. One day, back when I was at my heaviest, I went outside to run and I couldn't even run at a slow pace for a minute. I was getting too tired. That threw me because I have a military background and I was used to being in very good physical condition. I used to be able to go for five or six miles, no problem. When I realized that I couldn't run without stopping to catch my breath, I knew I was way off track.

So in addition to changing the way I ate, I also started walking for exercise. Then I slowly started running. I built myself back up. Now I work out four to five times a week, running, walking, and weight training.

It took me three to four weeks to start eating completely healthy. I had gotten so into the junk food that if I saw someone with a bag of chips or candy, I'd literally start to shake. It was like my body was going through some type of withdrawal. I really was an addict with junk food. It had become such a part of life. Sugar-free gum helped a lot. When I had the desire to eat junk food, I'd chew gum instead. That helped take the edge off.

I also began breaking up my meals throughout the day, and I still do. I have a mini meal every two to three hours so I never get hungry. All in all, it took me about four months to lose the weight and I've maintained my current weight since 1994.

You want to hear something funny? I saw my little cousin recently—the one who made that "fat" comment. Of course, she's older now. Anyway, she saw me and said, "Dot, you look so small!" and asked how I did it. I told her that I had to learn one very important thing: It's a lifestyle.

I love to eat and I don't like the concept of deprivation. I knew I had to do one of two things: either be heavy and have low energy or exercise and eat right. Eating right was the hardest part for me. Since I'd been bingeing so much, it was difficult for me to adopt a healthy way of eating. That's why it has to be a lifestyle change instead of a quick fix. It's easier to do if you know you can eat the treats you love now and then. Not every day, but once in a while.

Don't get me wrong. You do have to get real about food. I came up in a family that ate lots of fatty foods, lots of greasy foods. Nowadays, when I fix cabbage I steam it, and my family thinks that's just the nastiest thing in the world. I love fried chicken, but I know I can't eat it every day. It's about learning how to cook old favorites in new ways.

Not too long ago, I went to a relative's house for dinner and the biggest part of the meal was meat and potatoes. I asked her, "Where are the vegetables?" And she said, "We've got French fries."

Just last Christmas, my family was all together for the holidays. My sister's a wonderful cook and she had all the greens made the traditional way. So I told her I was going to get some lettuce and tomatoes and make myself a salad. She just looked at me and said, "We have vegetables, Dorothy."

I love greens and all that stuff; I do come from a Southern background, after all. I'm not saying I'm going to give that up, but I have to manage my new lifestyle, which means preparing my foods differently. Now, I may not pull that fix-my-own-salad-stuff in my mother's house, or try to tell her how to make her food. Come on, you know I can't go home and say something like, "Honey, there's too much grease up in here" to my *mother*. But I can ask her to go walking with me. And I can talk to her about health and fitness—which I do.

For any sister trying to lose weight, it's so important to love yourself for who you are, whether you're a size 10 or 20. A lot of times we have this distorted reality of what size we should be. A healthy mind-set is one that says whether you're a size 8, 10, 12, or 22, you're going to love your body. Take care of you. Go get your nails done, keep your feet done, buy a beautiful outfit, eat well, if you can't run then walk. You know what I'm saying? Be good to yourself regardless of how much you want to lose.

Once you do that, then try to look at health and fitness as a lifestyle, not a cure-all for getting into a size 6. It should simply be about wanting to be healthy and feeling good. When I first started losing weight, I was in that mirror every day and on that scale every day. If the numbers went up a little bit I'd get so depressed. What I learned to do is look at the whole picture and not so much at my size or my pounds. Think about the positives you achieve each day: *I drank six glasses of water today. I exercised today. I ate vegetables with my lunch and dinner today.* And so on.

Know that your weight can fluctuate. If the scale was my only criteria, I probably would have gone out and shot myself. But I made myself stay off the scale and I used a tape measure instead. I put red stars on my calendar to indicate that I'd done my workout for the day. After a while I stopped worrying about it.

You need to eliminate what I call the all-or-nothing attitude. That's when you think, "Oh God, I ate a piece of chocolate cake. That's it. It's over." And then you start eating everything in the world. Or if you didn't have an opportunity to work out and you think, "I may as well not do anything." Instead, resolve to work out tomorrow, even if you just go outside and walk for 20 minutes.

We defeat ourselves sometimes by having an unrealistic mind-set. We put too much pressure on ourselves. I used to do that. But because I've given myself permission to do or not do, it has helped me maintain a healthy lifestyle. I don't get freaked out. This summer I picked up a few pounds because of all the cookouts. But it didn't keep me from doing my thing. I still walked and worked out. Bottom line: Don't beat yourself up over every little thing and don't compare yourself to other people.

Most important, sisters need to support each other. There's a black woman at my gym who's very heavy and I admire her so much. I saw her today and she was doing the weights. I nodded at her and spoke. When I left, I went over to her and said, "You have a good workout." We sisters have to give each other encouragement. I guess I'm just from the old school that way.

CHAPTER 2

⊗

Living Longer,
Living Better

We know you're eager to get started. You're feeling pumped—ready to shed those excess pounds and get fit. But before you re-do your menus or break out the Lycra, you need to understand the big picture. Remember, you're taking control of more than your eating and exercise habits; you're taking control of your life. We want you to stay focused on what's really important—that's the key to successfully changing your life for the better.

Take a moment, sit back and think about your family. Don't worry, you'll see where we're going with this in a minute. How many of your heavy female relatives have high blood pressure? How many have diabetes? What about heart problems? Are you one of them? The sad truth is that obesity is killing us, and the evidence is often right in our own living rooms. The sheer number of sisters in our communities who have died of or are suffering from obesity-related diseases should be enough of a wake-up call. But hypertension, heart disease, and diabetes are so prevalent among our elderly that many of us assume they are inevitable consequences of aging.

Let's get one thing straight right now. They're not inevitable. While it's true that heredity places you at higher risk, you still have the power to take control. Adopt a healthier lifestyle and you'll add years to your life.

To help you truly understand the huge impact weight has on health, we've put together a straightforward primer of the most common—and serious—obesity-related health problems African-American women face. Seeing the possible consequences of being overweight in front of you will do two things. First, it will help you focus on the real reason for us to get fit—our health. Second, it will keep you motivated. Simply reread this chapter whenever willpower wanes, to remind yourself that every pound you lose equals a longer, better, more active life.

Heart Disease

What is it?

Heart disease is damage to the heart caused by a narrowing or blockage of the coronary arteries that supply the heart with blood. When the blood supply is severely reduced or cut off altogether, the result is a myocardial infarction—more commonly known as a heart attack.

What can it do?

Heart attacks can cause death or long-term heart complications. Heart attack survivors have an increased chance of suffering another one in coming years.

What are the symptoms?

Sudden chest pain that radiates down the left arm or to the jaw and the back, shortness of breath, clammy skin, nausea, profuse sweating, weakness, possible vomiting.

Many people who've suffered heart attacks have a history of angina pectoris, dull chest pain usually brought on by physical exertion and relieved by a few minutes of rest. If you've ever felt that way after, say, climbing a few flights of stairs, take it seriously. It's a red flag that your heart isn't getting enough blood and oxygen.

How does it affect black women and how does weight play a role?

More sisters in this country die from heart disease than from any other disease. In fact, between the ages of 34 and 74, we have a 38 percent higher chance of suffering a fatal heart attack than Caucasian women do, according to the American Heart Association.

There's no question that weight is a crucial factor. Obesity increases blood cholesterol and triglyceride levels, which ups the risk of heart disease; decreases HDL, the "good" cholesterol linked with lower risk; and raises blood pressure, which experts cite as a major contributor to heart attacks.

Diabetes

What is it?

Called "sugar" by many black folks, diabetes mellitus is a disease that occurs when the body is not able to use glucose (a form of sugar) as it should. Normally, the pancreas produces insulin, the hormone responsible for converting glucose into energy. With diabetes, too little or no insulin is produced, or what is produced is ineffective. As a result, the level of glucose in the blood becomes abnormally high, leading to a variety of health problems.

There are two main types of diabetes mellitus: insulin-dependent (Type I) and noninsulin-dependent (Type II). In Type I, the pancreas doesn't make any insulin, or it makes virtually none. This type, which usually occurs suddenly, most commonly starts in people under the age of thirty, quite often between the ages of ten and sixteen. Type I diabetes typically requires daily injections of insulin.

In Type II, the pancreas produces some insulin, but either it's not enough to meet the body's needs, or the body isn't able to use it effectively. Type II usually develops more gradually, most often in people over the age of forty, and accounts for 90 to 95 percent of all diabetes cases. Unfortunately, many people aren't even aware that they have it. Although injections aren't required to control Type II diabetes, a change in diet and exercise is necessary.

What can it do?

If left untreated, diabetes can cause serious complications, including blindness, kidney failure, nervous system disorder (impaired sensation or pain in the feet and hands), amputations (typically of lower limbs), and even death.

What are the symptoms?

Excessive urination, extreme thirst, constant hunger, unexplained weight loss, fatigue, blurred vision, tingling and numbness in hands and feet, itching, slow healing of sores.

How does it affect black women and does weight play a role?

Type II diabetes is especially common among black women. One in four sisters age fifty-five and older has the disease, according to the National Institute of Diabetes and Digestive and Kidney Diseases (NIDDK). What's more, African-Americans with diabetes are more likely to develop complications than are their white counterparts. Consider these findings from the NIDDK: Sisters are three times more likely to become blind from diabetes than white women; blacks are up to five times more likely to experience diabetes-related kidney failure; and African-Americans undergo more lower-extremity amputations.

Aside from heredity, obesity and physical inactivity are two of the biggest risk factors for Type II diabetes in black women. Recent research from the NIDDK shows that the location of excess weight may play a role in the likelihood of developing the disease. While obesity in and of itself puts us at high risk, it seems upper body obesity is an even greater risk factor for Type II diabetes than extra pounds below the waist. Since African-American women have a tendency to gain the bulk of our excess weight above the belt, our chances of developing Type II is increased that much more. And because we lead a more sedentary lifestyle than white women do, we lose a strong protective factor against diabetes—physical activity.

High Blood Pressure

What is it?

Hypertension, or high blood pressure as it is more often called, is a condition in which resting blood pressure is consistently raised. A blood pressure reading of 120/80 is considered normal. The first number refers to systolic pressure, the maximum force placed on your arteries as blood surges through with each heartbeat. The second number is diastolic pressure, the lowest pressure placed on arteries when the heart is relaxed between beats. A high systolic pressure means your arteries and your heart are being strained every time the heart pumps blood. A high diastolic pressure means your blood vessels barely have a chance to rest.

It's normal for blood pressure to go up when you're physically active or under stress. With hypertension, however, pressure stays up, even when you're at your most relaxed.

What can it do?

Uncontrolled hypertension can be deadly, causing stroke, heart failure, and kidney damage.

What are the symptoms?

High blood pressure is called "the silent killer" for good reason—it has no symptoms and often goes undetected. That's why it's so important to have your pressure checked every time you visit the doctor.

How does it affect black women and how does weight play a role?

According to the National Center for Health Statistics, nearly a third of all black women have high blood pressure. And the American Heart Association estimates that one in five of us with the disease die from it each year.

Heredity, age, and race are all contributing factors: Black folks get it more often than whites, it tends to occur after age 35, and it usually runs in families. We can't control these things. But we can control our weight and it's crucial that we do. Years of research shows that obesity significantly increases the risk of developing hypertension.

Stroke

What is it?

A stroke occurs when blood vessels to the brain burst or clog. When the affected part of the brain doesn't get the flow of blood it needs, it becomes damaged, at which point any body functions controlled by that region of the brain become impaired.

There are three types of stroke: cerebral thrombosis, cerebral embolism, and hemorrhage. The most common type of stroke is a cerebral thrombosis, which is blockage by a clot that has built up on the wall of a brain artery. Cerebral embolism occurs when an artery is blocked by a clot that has been swept in by the bloodstream. A hemorrhage happens when a blood vessel in or near the brain ruptures and bleeding occurs in the brain or over its surface.

What can it do?

About one-third of strokes are fatal. Nonlethal strokes can cause paralysis or diminished capacity on one side of the body, and impaired language and speech.

What are the symptoms?

Headache, dizziness, slurred speech, difficulty swallowing, trouble seeing.

How does it affect black women and how does weight play a role?

According to the American Heart Association, more than twenty-five hundred African-American women were killed by strokes in 1996. The fact is, we are nearly three times more likely to die of one than are white women. Because hypertension and diabetes are two factors that greatly increase our chances of suffering a stroke, weight ups the odds—and not in our favor. Being severely overweight makes you twice as likely to have one.

Breast Cancer

What is it?

All cancer stems from abnormal cells that grow and spread rapidly. In the case of breast cancer, the abnormal cells form a malignant tumor in the breast.

What can it do?

Breast cancer can be fatal, most often when it is detected late, after it has already spread to other parts of the body. Regular self-examination and mammograms are essential to catch the disease in its early stages.

Many women who are diagnosed with breast cancer do not have to undergo a radical mastectomy, in which the entire breast, chest muscles, and lymph nodes are removed. Many surgeons today recommend a lumpectomy—removal of only the cancerous tissue.

What are the symptoms?

Usually a lump is felt during self-examination or a doctor's visit. There may also be dark discharge from the nipple, indentation of the nipple, and dimpled skin over the site of the lump.

How does it affect black women and how does weight play a role?

Breast cancer is the most common form of cancer in black women. White women are more apt to get it, but we're more likely to die from it—twice as likely, in fact. Sisters have the highest mortality and lowest survival rates for the disease, according to the National Cancer Institute. Late detection is the primary reason for our lower survival rate. Typically, by the time we are diagnosed with breast cancer, it has already spread. Some studies also suggest that tumor cells grow faster in black women, leading to a more aggressive cancer.

No one knows for sure what causes breast cancer or whether one factor contributes more than another, but extensive research does show a definite link to obesity. One possible explanation for the connection is increased estrogen production; studies have found a greater incidence of breast cancer in women with excessively high estrogen levels. If you are one of the many sisters who rely on estrogen-replacement therapy—which can protect us from heart disease and other illnesses, not to mention help ease the way through menopause—discuss the possible estrogen/breast cancer connection with your doctor.

Being severely overweight can also adversely affect breast cancer detection since small tumors may be harder to diagnose.

Cervical Cancer

What is it?

Cancer of the cervix, the lower part of the uterus, occurs in two main forms: squamous cell carcinoma, the most common type, which is often associated with the human papillomavirus (the cause of genital warts), and adenocarcinoma, which is much more rare. Cervical cancer stems from abnormal changes in the cells on the surface of the cervix. This precancerous stage is known as cervical dysplasia. Sometimes dysplasia goes away all by itself, never leading to cancer. But no woman should rely on that happening since cervical cancer is one of the most common cancers affecting women.

What can it do?

If untreated, it can spread to other pelvic organs. Although cervical cancer can be fatal, the disease is highly curable if detected early.

What are the symptoms?

Precancerous stages have no symptoms. Malignancy, however, may eventually cause unexplained vaginal bleeding and pain in the pelvic region. A simple Pap smear can detect cervical abnormalities, both in precancerous and cancerous stages.

How does it affect black women and how does weight play a role?

The odds of a sister developing cervical cancer are greater than they are for a Caucasian woman. Black women are three times as likely to get the disease and twice as likely to die from it, according to the American Cancer Society.

Though experts can't say exactly how obesity puts a woman at greater risk, many studies show that overweight women do, in fact, have higher rates of cervical cancer.

Endometrial Cancer

What is it?

Endometrial cancer, also caller uterine cancer, occurs when malignant growth develops in the lining of the uterus.

What can it do?

Endometrial cancer can kill, but if caught and treated in its early stages, survival rates are very good. If the disease spreads, cancer cells may be carried through the bloodstream or lymph nodes in the pelvis and abdomen.

What are the symptoms?

Prior to menopause, the symptoms of endometrial cancer include unusually heavy menstrual periods, or vaginal bleeding in between periods or following sex. After menopause, a blood-stained vaginal discharge is the most common symptom.

Abnormal bleeding doesn't always indicate endometrial cancer; several other conditions could be the culprit. If you do experience any of these symptoms, though, you should have it checked out by your doctor.

Pap smears aren't considered reliable tests for endometrial cancer because they may not detect abnormal cells. A biopsy or a D&C (dilatation and curettage) is much more accurate since both methods allow testing of an actual sample of the uterine lining.

The most common treatment for early-stage endometrial cancer is hysterectomy and removal of the fallopian tubes and ovaries.

How does it affect black women and how does weight play a role?

Of the estimated twenty-one hundred black women who developed endometrial cancer in 1996, nearly half of them died. African-American women are more likely to be diagnosed with the disease at later stages than are white women, and we're at least 15 percent less likely to survive, according to the American Cancer Society.

As with breast cancer, research suggests that endometrial cancer is tied to excess estrogen and that obesity contributes to the disease by significantly raising estrogen levels. Being very heavy also cuts down a black woman's chance for survival. Hypertension and diabetes, conditions highly prevalent among sisters, are both factors in endometrial cancer death.

Osteoarthritis

What is it?

Osteoarthritis is a common form of arthritis that's caused by wear and tear on the joints; healthy cartilage lining the joints deteriorates, and outgrowths of new bone, called osteophytes, may form, producing a gnarled appearance. This joint disease typically affects the knees, hands, hips, back, and neck.

What can it do?

Osteoarthritis can cause pain, swelling, and stiffness, making everyday activities such as walking and getting dressed difficult, and may eventually lead to severe disability.

What are the symptoms?

Typical symptoms include pain, tenderness, and swelling in the joints.

How does it affect black women and how does weight play a role?

Osteoarthritis affects scores of African-American women, especially as we age. Research shows that the more overweight you are, the more likely you are to develop the disease, especially in the knees. It stands to reason that carrying excess pounds puts more stress on your body's lower-extremity joints. While the same logic may not apply to osteoarthritis in the hands, studies suggest that a particular hormone may be the link between obesity and this type of osteoarthritis.

Sister to Sister
XOXOXOXOX

Gail Alston, a forty-one-year-old banking applications examiner from New York, New York
Current weight: 170 pounds
Amount lost: 20 pounds

A few years ago I was having family problems and I was under a lot of stress. I turned to food to deal with the pressure. Junk food was my thing—pastries, ice cream, potato chips. I'd snack at lunchtime and again at night while watching television. I couldn't even look at the TV without munching on some Lay's potato chips.

There was a time in my life when if I'd put on a few pounds, I'd simply ease up on my eating and I would lose the weight within a couple of days. But when these family problems started, that wasn't happening anymore. I'd eat and the weight would stay. It wasn't like I packed it on all at once, though. The pounds came on gradually over six years.

What made me finally take action after six years? I started feeling bad physically. I'd get light-headed and dizzy at times, and that scared me. Then my sister was diagnosed with weight-related diabetes. That was a big wake-up call for me. I became very concerned about my own health. I didn't want that to happen to me, so I stepped on the scale to see how much I weighed. I hadn't been on a scale in I don't know how long and I had no clue how much I truly weighed. I wasn't interested in facing reality, you know. I had pushed the scale under the bed ages ago and left it there. When I finally dragged it out and stepped on it, I actually looked over my shoulder for a split second as if to see who'd stepped on with me. I thought, "This can't be all me" as I read the numbers: 190 pounds.

I looked at losing weight as a challenge. A challenge I could win. I didn't want anything to happen to me, health-wise, so I made up my mind to deal with the situation.

The first thing I did was stop going to the supermarket, literally. I sent my son instead. He's twenty-one and still liv-ing at home, so I let him do the grocery shopping. I told him what to buy and I knew I could trust him to make good food choices. My son is very lean and in good shape, so I knew he'd pick healthy things. Plus he knew what I liked and what I needed, so, for example, even though he drinks whole milk, he bought skim milk for me. I just thought it would be easier in the beginning to let him take care of the shopping.

Basically, I ate less. I really paid attention to portion sizes, and had lots of salads, fish, and chicken. I didn't cook the way I used to; I tried to make my meals healthier. I also made lunch the biggest meal of the day and kept my dinners light. I stopped eating after 8:30 P.M., too.

I've tried to make food secondary. Boy, I can remember times when I'd wake up in the morning and immediately start preplanning my meals for the entire day. "What am I going to have for breakfast? What am I going to have for lunch? What am I going to have for dinner?" It was obses-sive. I had to change my way of thinking.

Over the years, I'd work out off and on, nothing consis-tent. But once I made up my mind to lose weight, I began exercising regularly. I tried to do a variety of activities— and still do. I play racquetball, walk, do step aerobics and Tae-bo. I work out three times a week for 90 minutes each time.

Staying away from junk food has been the hardest part for me. Two months after I started my new lifestyle, I bought myself a coffee-almond ice-cream bar. Häagen-Dazs no less. I hadn't had any junk food in all that time. Girl, it was like heaven. I didn't beat myself up about it, though. I enjoyed every bite. But I knew I wasn't going to get another one the next day. Instead I'd be right back out there working up a sweat. I wasn't going to allow one indulgence to get the better of me. In order to keep myself in check I think about how much I've accomplished so far and remind myself that I don't want to sabotage all of my good efforts.

I'm currently trying to lose another 20 to 25 pounds and I have confidence that I will do it. I'm going to stay motivated. I have to. I've come too far to stop now. I have to do this for my health. It's not a vanity thing.

I do wish more sisters were out there exercising and getting healthy. I don't see enough of us when I'm working out. Last summer I ran in Central Park—it was another of my exercise activities. Now, you can literally see hundreds of people running and jogging in Central Park. You know how many sisters I saw during the whole summer? Less than ten. I was like, "Where are the sisters?"

We have to move our bodies. I am serious. If you're having a hard time at thirty and forty, what's going to happen to you at fifty and sixty? If I could say one thing to sisters who are out there trying to lose weight and get healthy, it would be, "Never give up." If you get to a point where you start thinking, "Forget this," that's okay. Tomorrow's a new day. Just keep going.

CHAPTER 3

Why We're Unique

Pretty eye-opening, right? You may have known about the relationship between high blood pressure and weight, but were you aware of the diabetes link? How about the cancer connection? If you're like most sisters, it probably came as a shock. Therein lies the problem. Too many of us don't realize how much we are risking by toting these extra pounds around.

Well, you're ahead of the game now. Since you've already made a commitment to yourself to shed weight, you're going to boost your health. We know you might be thinking, "Well, if I realize what I need to do, why can't I just head down to the nearest Weight Watchers meeting or sweat it out at a local gym like everybody else? Why do I need my own special program?" Because you're not like everyone else. When it comes to weight loss, sisters are different. Our bodies work differently; our minds and spirits need different motivations.

We'd like you to try something. Close your eyes and imagine two women—one black, the other white—standing side by side. Both of them are overweight. Who do you think needs to lose the most weight? Odds are, the sister is heavier.

Research tells us that, on average, African-American women

weigh more than their white counterparts. The question is why. If we examine those two women the answers become clear. By just standing there, their bodies are burning calories. It's what experts call resting energy expenditure, or basal metabolic rate. Simply put, it's the number of calories your body burns when you're doing absolutely nothing. Surprisingly, the body eats up roughly two-thirds of our daily calories when we are just lounging around. Unfortunately for black women, on average we burn nearly one hundred fewer calories at rest each day than white women do, according to a study from the University of Pennsylvania. Researchers there, led by Dr. Gary D. Foster, wanted to find out if biology could help explain why obesity is more prevalent among black women than white women, and why black women have a harder time losing weight. Indeed, their study found that obese sisters burned about 1,638 calories a day at rest, while white women burned 1,731 calories. Even after adjustments were made for body weight and muscle mass, the study's conclusion remained the same.

These findings suggest that black and white women are, in fact, built differently. It would be so easy to blame everything on biology, wouldn't it? You know how that would go: "Oh girl, it's so hard for me to lose weight, what with this slow metabolism and all." But that's a cop-out. The truth is, biology is just one piece of the puzzle.

Gathering 'Round the Table

We've already talked about how our culture helps keep us fat. A big woman is more accepted in our community; we don't feel the same pressure as white women do to be stick-thin. We have a strong, positive self-image—one that allows us to feel good about ourselves no matter our size.

But take a closer look at black folks' social structure. Peel back the layers and you'll uncover a tradition that nurtures our soul on one hand, while unwittingly compromising our health on the other. Ours is a social structure based on family and community, on sharing and cooperation—all blessings to be sure. But because our traditional ways of interacting with one another often center around food—typically high-fat, high-calorie food—we have a tendency to focus less on the health consequences of what we eat and more on simply enjoying our loved ones.

We can't deny that food brings our people together. For us, it's not about how many calories are in that heaping helping of macaroni and cheese or how much fat is dripping off of those tender neckbones. It's about laughing, talking, and loving over a good meal. And we're not about to give up that kinship; the roots go too deep. Our African ancestors lived by a deeply-held belief in community. Tribal celebrations centered around the harvest and the people. Fellowship and family ties were honored at every meal. There was no such thing as the individual; there was only the group.

Indeed, it was this sense of family, of connection, of belonging to a loving group, that sustained our ancestors when they were brought to these shores as slaves. Though separated from blood ties, they survived by building new bonds of kinship. Over hundreds of years our sense of community and connection has thrived, and the food-based celebrations that united us in the past continue to do so today.

Even in times of crisis we pull together by way of food. If a family in our community falls on hard times, they can count on neighbors to bring over a plate of this and a dish of that to see them through. It is our sharing tradition, our communal heritage, that brings us all 'round the table as one. No, we are never going to give that up. Nor should we. It's one of the wonderful characteristics that define us as a people. However, we need to rethink what we're putting on the table and how we're preparing it. If we don't, we are never going to get a handle on our health

Sisterfriends Make All the Difference

As much as our social customs color the way we share food with kin, they may also color our success or failure in traditional weight loss programs. How? Let's go back to those two women for a moment. The white woman who's overweight can join a standard weight-loss program and successfully drop pounds by simply adhering to the behavior-modification principles of the program. The overweight sister, however, is apt to have a far more difficult time making that program work for her.

Several studies, including research by University of Illinois psychologist Shiriki Kumanyika, Ph.D., suggest that typical weight-loss programs are based on white, male values and motivations, specifically self-direction, competition, autonomy, and self-motivation. When a woman joins one of these programs, she is given some sort of food plan, information on proper food groups, portion sizes and fat/calorie content, exercise suggestions and the like, then sent on her merry way. It's up to her to make the program work. Sure, there are weekly meetings with other members, perhaps even one-on-one counseling with a staff professional. But, in the end, the onus is on the woman who joined to succeed or fail.

The goal of these programs is to help you change your behavior. The problem for us is that this self-management style of weight loss just doesn't mesh with our values. Our history shows that we are a cooperative, group-oriented people. Our motivations are fed by strong support systems. We don't know the other women in these programs. They don't have a vested interest in our success. It's all about the individual. A sister is more likely to reach her weight-loss goal when she has a caring, supportive group of family and friends around to cheer her on—or better yet, who are actively persuing the same get-fit goals.

When we join one of these programs, our expectations may be vastly different from those of the white woman sitting next to us at a meeting. We yearn for the "we're all in it together" feeling that we get from those who are closest to us. When you know there's someone out there going through the same things you are, someone you can call any time to talk through the rough spots— say, snack attacks at midnight or the struggle to make favorite soul dishes more healthful—it helps. But are we going to drop in on other program members we really don't know, whom we've just met, or pick up the phone to call them? Are we going to do that with a staff counselor who we see once a week, who leads tons of other groups just like ours? No, we're not. We're going to stick it out alone, just like the program suggests we do. We're going to keep trying to convince ourselves that we can do this without out anyone's help.

Why put yourself through that? Yes, you do have it in you to reach your goal. You can shed however many pounds you need to in order to improve your health. All we're saying is there's a better way to go about it—one that offers you the type of support you require. Our cultural differences don't have to present an impossible roadblock to weight-loss success. We believe there are two positive, spirit-fortifying ways for sisters to get fit that tap into our long history of community, kinship, sharing, and group motivation. One is what we like to call a "sister circle," and the other is the church.

Starting your own sister circle is one of the easiest and most satisfying things you can do. A common goal and a promise to support one another is all it takes to create one. Gather together several of your girlfriends—the ones who have decided to shed pounds to improve their health as you have—and agree to do it together. We'll do the rest. The best foods, the healthier soul food menus, the core exercise program, the stay-psyched tips—we'll provide those for you in these pages. You simply have to share it all with your girls. How easy is that? You share everything with them anyway, right?

One important thing to keep in mind, though: You all have to be committed to doing this as a group. You are a team, a solid unit. That will be the key to your success. Remember, the purpose of the sister circle is to provide the support and continuous encouragement that you can't find in a standard weight-loss program.

Okay, so your girls are down with the idea. Everyone's excited and ready to go. First things first. You've got to set some ground rules. You didn't think the sister circle was going to be a catch-as-catch-can operation, did you? Sure, you're going to have fun doing this together, but you need a bit of structure for it to work well.

That said, all of you should decide upon a meeting schedule. Once a week, twice a week—whatever feels right for the group. Think about your meeting place, too. Do you always want to have them at your house? Someone else's house? Do you want to rotate? Who's married or living with someone? Who has kids? How will their schedules coincide with the sister circle's meeting schedule? All of these factors need to be ironed out upfront.

What will your meetings consist of? Do you want there to be a hard-and-fast itinerary, or do you want to keep things loose? Perhaps you want to use the time to simply talk about how things are going for everyone. Who's having a hard time? What are the problem areas? What type of solutions can the group come up with to help out?

You may want to set aside time to discuss food in-depth. Who has a great low-calorie recipe for cornbread? Who found a tasty low-fat substitute for seasoning greens? (Don't forget to check out Appendix B for this sort of useful information.)

You might even want to designate a few minutes for positive affirmations—sayings and words of wisdom to help you all stay focused and committed. Share them with the group. Recite them out loud. Often some meaningful inner work goes a long way toward helping us reach our goals.

It's up to you and your sisterfriends to decide how you want to spend your meeting time. Get input from everyone—you should each have a voice. Working it out together will give your sister circle a closer connection.

Also be sure to brainstorm ways to touch base outside of your regular meetings. This is crucial. If you need to pick up the phone when motivation wanes, you want to know that your girl on the other end of the line will be there for you with just the right "you can do it" words of encouragement. Say you have five friends in your sister circle. Perhaps you all agree to take turns calling each person two or three times a week just to see how everything's going. Or you might decide to divvy up "on call" duty for those times when one or more of you needs extra support. This is the sort of intimate, anytime-anywhere caring that you just won't find in a traditional weight-loss program. Come up with your own terms and stick with them.

Figure out a feasible workout schedule too. We'll get to the exercises in the next chapter, just keep in mind that doing them as a group can make all the difference. Imagine the fun you'll have sweating it out with your sister circle while some funky R&B plays in the background. Who needs a gym full of strangers when you can push back the coffee table and get to work with your friends? You'll have privacy, camaraderie, your choice of music, your own timetable, your own bathroom to shower in, and the $500 or $600 you would have spent otherwise.

Consider designating one night a week as party night, girls' night out, whatever you want to call it. Grab your sisters and hit the clubs. Getting your groove on counts as exercise too, you know. The workout we provide in chapter 4 is just part of the exercise package. Find ways to make fitness fun and you'll be more apt to stick with it. Having your girls along for the ride—bike ride, that is—will definitely make it more enjoyable. Here's a perfect opportunity to let your inner child loose. When's the last time you played a game of Frisbee? How about jump rope? We bet you spent many a hazy summer afternoon jumping double dutch with your friends. Why not do it again? See if your sister circle can still last ten minutes without messing up the rope, like they did when they were little. Here's another idea for you: Challenge your girls to a bit of in-line skating. Never tried it before? Take lessons together. All of these ideas are creative, fun, kid-in-you ways to break a sweat. Trust us, if you get your sister circle hooked on these sorts of workouts in addition to the core exercise and walking routine coming up in the next chapter, you'll have a blast burning off that fat.

Getting with the Spirit

Your church is another great avenue for shaping up. Think about it. You will have love, support, encouragement, and kinship, all under one spiritual roof. Most likely, your church already offers some sort of community health screening. You can easily take that one step further and start a fitness/wellness program. Even if your house of worship doesn't offer health screenings, you can still organize a weight-loss program there. We explain how in Appendix A.

Skeptical about whether a church-based weight-loss program can work for you? Consider the case of the Baltimore Church High Blood Pressure Program. Dr. Shiriki Kumanyika took an in-depth look at this program to discover the keys to its success. Her findings prove that a church-based setting can help a great many sisters shed pounds for good.

The Baltimore program, officially called Lose Weight and Win, began in 1979 as a means of bringing together churches in Baltimore's black community to offer hypertension screenings and related health services. In 1984 an eight-week weight-control program was added to the mix. Two-hour meetings were held at each church once a week, and consisted of private weigh-ins, blood-pressure checks, discussions with a dietitian, a group meeting, and finally, an exercise session.

At the beginning of the program, each person set a weight-loss goal for the course of the eight weeks that could be no more than sixteen pounds. There was no prescribed diet plan; members ate what they usually did, but learned how to reduce fat and calories and to control portion sizes. They also kept food diaries—a wonderful tool for tracking when, what, and how much you eat. Seeing it all spelled out helps you identify trouble spots and trigger foods.

The Lose Weight and Win group meetings were the heart of the program. Everyone shared their experiences, brainstormed possible solutions for members' problems, and discussed goals and strategies. Here was where participants could find sincere support from people they knew, people they worshipped with every Sunday. Sharing that spiritual connection made them much more invested in everyone's success.

The exercise sessions of low-impact aerobics ran for a half hour to 45 minutes. In addition to this weekly workout, members were encouraged to break a sweat at least two more times each week.

The cost of this comprehensive program? A mere eight dollars, and anyone who couldn't pay was still welcomed to join. As an incentive, the membership money was pooled and awarded to the three people closest to their goal at the end of the eight weeks. Other incentives of the program included weekly prizes that members could use along the way, such as measuring cups and food scales. However, these weekly motivational prizes were not based on pounds lost, but on behavioral milestones reached.

In the end, a whopping 90 percent of the sisters in the program lost weight. We believe the methods and principles utilized in the Baltimore churches' Lose Weight and Win program can be replicated in other churches—like your church. Many of the behavior-modification techniques are similar to those used in traditional weight-loss programs, but the difference here is the religious and spiritual setting and the support it provides.

There is a collective identity within the black church, one that offers us strength and support— two things we need in order to win the weight war. If you had a weight-loss program available in your house of worship, you'd have continual access to other sisters who share your goals and who care deeply about whether or not you attain them. Every time you go to choir rehearsal, or Sunday service, or the church bazaar, or a prayer meeting, or a church supper, you'll be surrounded by the women in your weight-loss group, women with whom you share a spiritually-based history. You're comfortable with these sisters; you're among your peers. The church environment offers you a sense of peace and relaxation. It allows you to truly focus on what you're trying to accomplish. What better setting is there for your journey?

Sister to Sister
✕◆✕✕◆✕✕◆✕

Janice Nesbit, a thirty-eight-year-old accountant from Queens, New York
Current weight: 200 pounds
Amount lost: 40 pounds

My weight had escalated in the last three years, basically from inactivity. I never really saw myself as big. Sometimes we heavy sisters think that as long as we carry ourselves nice, we can carry the weight. And I was able to do that. I still received the same kind of positive attention at 240 pounds that I did when I was thinner. So I didn't think it of it as a negative. Yes, I felt uncomfortable at that weight, but I didn't look at it as some sort of downfall. Then I saw a picture of myself. I was dressed really nice, wearing a suit, the whole nine. But when I looked at myself I couldn't believe it. Because the black community is so accepting of weight, we often don't perceive how heavy we are. What's so sad about it is that our eating habits will kill us. The more I thought about it, the more I knew I had to make a change. In December 1997 I began.

At first I joined a gym for a year, but I only lost 12 pounds. I'm not really good about going to the gym. For me to get dressed, do my hair and makeup, go to work, hit the gym at lunchtime, then shower, redo my hair and makeup, get dressed all over again—oh, please! I only have an hour for lunch. I don't have time for all that. I think that's why I only lost 12 pounds in a year. It's a lot easier for me to work out at home. I can just roll out of bed, put on my workout gear, and get started. So I canceled my gym membership, bought a treadmill, and lost 40 pounds.

When I woke up in the morning, exercise was automatic and there were no distractions.

I got the idea for a treadmill from a friend of mine who's a fitness trainer. He used to tell me about this woman at his gym who started out as a size 20. He said she'd come to the gym every day, get on the treadmill for 30 minutes, stretch, then leave. That's all she did. My friend said this woman literally disappeared before his eyes. I figured I could do the same thing.

So I went out and bought a treadmill. I'd wake up at 5:30 every morning, have a light breakfast of fruit and toast, then I'd get on the treadmill for 30 to 45 minutes. Some mornings I'd do 15 to 30 minutes of an aerobics tape afterward, depending on how much time I had.

I know some sisters don't like to work out because of their hair. I can understand that, because I sweat profusely. I mean, dripping like a rain forest. When I first started exercising, I'd wash my hair in the shower after my workout. Then I'd pull it back in a ponytail to dry naturally. My hair broke off very badly as a result of always being back in a ponytail while wet. Well, I didn't want to worry about my hair breaking or sweating out so I cut it off. I sacrificed my hair to get my health back. I have a perm, but my hair is cut very short. Now I wash my hair every day after working out, slick it back with some gel, and go. Sometimes I go to the hair salon and get it done, you know, curled. But for the most part this is my look. It's very convenient for working out.

When I first started exercising I was extremely disciplined. I felt that if I didn't get up and work out, it would be even harder for me to get up the next day. The only time I had difficulty was on the weekends. I'd get up and put on my workout clothes, but many times I didn't get on the treadmill until noon—if at all—because I was doing things around the house. I'd tell myself, "I'll get to it. I just want to do this first." I learned that I can't do that because I'll end up not working out. I have to get up and get it over with. It definitely takes a lot of discipline.

That's why it's so important to find a workout that suits your personality. Otherwise you won't stick with it. I know me and I know how I am. I can't walk outside. I get distracted and I can't concentrate. If I see someone I know, I'll stop to talk. So it's better for me to exercise indoors.

As far as eating goes, it was pretty easy for me to make the transition to healthier habits because I like low-calorie foods anyway. I cut back on fat and I found alternatives to the junk food I was eating. I love ice cream. So I simply substituted for it with frozen yogurt. I began baking and grilling my foods. I ate lots of salads and vegetables. I'd carry around a bag of fresh vegetables in my purse—cucumbers, carrots, and carrot sticks. When I felt like munching, I'd just pull them out. I also kept a bottle of water handy. I'll tell you, drinking eight glasses of water a day was the hardest thing for me.

After a while, I found that I didn't really miss the junk food, the fried food, or the red meat. Eating well and exercising made me feel so much better. I didn't want that stuffed, sluggish feeling that I used to get from eating foods that were too heavy.

As I lost weight, friends kept asking me how I was doing it. Pretty soon, most of my girlfriends had gone out and bought treadmills too. I guess I motivated them.

It took me about six months to lose 40 pounds. I went from a size 18 to a 14. But I still want to lose 30 more pounds, so I'm making adjustments to my workout. I'd gone from every day to three days a week, but I'm going to go back up to five or six days a week. And I'm about to start kickboxing. I enjoy walking on the treadmill—I put on my headphones and listen to house music; it really gets me pumped up—but after a while you do get bored with the same routine. I want to do something to break it up a bit and lose the rest of this weight.

I want to be as healthy as I can be. My daughter always says, "Mommy, you think you're fat, but you're not." And I say to her, "Honey, I'm overweight and I just want to be healthy. If that means losing weight, that's what I'm going to do." I'm getting fit for me.

I'm single and I do date, but that's not why I'm trying to get in shape. Even if the brothers don't care about us losing weight, if we know we need to do it for health reasons, then we have to do what we have to do.

There was a time when my self-esteem had decreased. I consider myself to be very confident, but I allowed my weight to affect my self-esteem. Back when I first started trying to lose weight and I'd joined that gym, I met a brother who worked there. I couldn't understand why he was trying to talk to me; I felt like the biggest thing in the gym. Once we started dating I said to him, "I don't understand why you're talking to me and calling me sexy and gorgeous. I'd think you'd be jumping on every little body that walked in here." He told me that he didn't like little women. When I was losing weight he was very supportive. In my dating experience I haven't encountered any negative vibes from the brothers out there. They always speak and want to get to know me. My weight is not a concern for them. Any brothers I've dated, weight has always been an issue for me but never for them.

I now realize that what I need to focus on is my health. We all know that being heavy is not healthy. There are so many things out there working against sisters, it's even more important for us to eat right and exercise because it will help bring us longevity. We have to do it for ourselves. We have to love ourselves.

CHAPTER 4

Work That Body!

If someone discovered a way for people to lose weight without having to move their butts off the couch, that person would be a millionaire. Everyone wants the quick fix, the easy solution. We're human, after all—not to mention busy. These days it seems sisters have precious little time for themselves. Work has us crazed, family is clamoring for our attention. Who in the world has time to exercise? You do! No, really. You *do*. There's no law requiring you to work out for thirty or sixty minutes straight. In fact, you can break it up into ten- or fifteen-minute chunks several times a day and still get the same health benefits. And trust us, the benefits are worth getting, especially if you're trying to shed pounds.

The bottom line is that you need to move your body if you want to lose weight—period. There's no two ways about it. Sure, you can probably drop a few pounds by drastically cutting your caloric intake. But sooner or later your body's going to rebel. And you know what that means. Those pounds are going to come back with a vengeance. Chances are, you'll end up weighing more than you did when you started out.

Think of your body as a car—it needs calories for fuel, for energy. It's how we keep going every day. If you cut way back on your calories, it's like depriving your car of the fuel it needs to run, only it's your body that's going to break down, not your wheels. In order to keep trucking along, your body will do whatever it takes to hold on to every single calorie you put in it. The less you eat, the more your metabolism slows down, making it harder and harder for you to lose weight.

So what's the key to revving up your engine, that is, your metabolism? You guessed it—exercise. Break a good sweat and your body won't be inclined to hang onto those calories at all costs. You'll burn them up, and not just during your workout. Research proves that vigorous exercise has an added bonus: afterburn. Your metabolism keeps running strong even after your workout is done, so you'll still be burning calories hours later. And that's good news for sisters like you who are ready to take charge of their health.

Lose the Excuses

The more you know about the relationship between exercise and good health, the more likely you'll be to make it a part of your daily routine. We're not saying you have to get out there and run a marathon (though if you feel pumped enough to give it a shot in a few months, more power to you girl!). All you have to do is find a way to incorporate at least thirty minutes of moderately intense exercise into your life most days of the week.

For many of us, that's asking a lot. The truth is, black folks tend to work out less frequently than whites, according to several studies, and that's one of the reasons sisters are more apt to be overweight than white women are. We don't want to spend our down-time pumping iron or taking a step class. We'd much rather relax. So says a recent Pennsylvania State College of Medicine study. Those surveyed feel that working out only adds stress to their already stressful and hectic lives. But if those folks would just devote ten or fifteen minutes to, say, a brisk walk, they would realize that exercise actually helps alleviate stress and tension.

Don't fall into the same trap. If you're still clinging to that tired, old "I don't have time" excuse, just let it go. You will benefit in so many ways—and we're not talking solely about losing weight, though that's way up on the list. Check out this rundown of workout wonders, then we'll see how those excuses hold up.

Regular exercise can:

- *Help prevent disease.* Physical activity boosts your cardiovascular health by strengthening your heart, lowering blood pressure, raising your HDL ("good") cholesterol levels, and lowering LDL ("bad") cholesterol levels, all of which help reduce the risk of heart attacks, according to the American Heart Association. Exercise also protects against stroke, hypertension, diabetes, osteoarthritis, and certain cancers.
- *Boost your immune system.* This is an important benefit because a strong immune system makes your body better able to fight off infections.
- *Increase stamina.* When you "work out" your heart and lungs on a regular basis, you give them more power to do their jobs well. You'll find that you have more energy, too.
- *Trim pounds.* If you combine fat-burning, muscle-building exercise with smart, healthy eating, you'll lose weight and keep it off.
- *Stave off osteoporosis.* As women age, we lose bone mass. But weight-bearing exercise, such as strength-training, walking, and running, can build bones, making them denser and stronger. Though white women are more prone to osteoporosis, sisters are still at risk for the disease, which thins and weakens bones, increasing one's susceptibility to fractures.
- *Increase muscle mass.* Since muscle burns calories, the more you have the better off you'll be. Strength levels will improve as well.
- *Relieve stress.* Exercise releases feel-good brain chemicals, such as endorphins and serotonin, which make you feel relaxed

and calm. Physical activity also gives you an outlet for the tension and anxiety of the day.

- *Lift your mood.* Workouts offer an array of psychological gifts: They reduce depression, boost self-esteem, and lift your spirits when you're feeling down.

- *Improve sleep.* Aerobic exercise is a great stress-buster, and less stress translates to better, sounder sleep. Just be sure to work out well before bedtime, though, or the increase in your adrenaline may keep you up.

- *Enhance sex.* Since regular exercise improves your cardio capacity, you'll have more stamina in bed. Working out also increases testosterone levels—yes, women have that hormone too—which means your sex drive will get a nudge up.

All of this equals better health for sisters. It's hard to argue with that kind of proof, isn't it? So give working out a go. Start off slowly and ease your way into it. Soon you'll be feeling the positive effects and wondering what took you so long to get into the groove.

That's how most sisters feel when they start an exercise program. They may be a little wary at first, coming up with all kinds of excuses, including that old standby, lack of time. We've heard them all. "I don't know how to lift weights." "I'm a klutz." "I don't want to sweat out my hair." "I don't have anyone to watch my kids." "I'm too embarrassed to set foot in a gym." And on and on. But as soon as they get into it, they love it because they start feeling better right away and begin seeing results in a matter of weeks.

Remember the Baltimore church program, Lose Weight and Win? The folks who took part evaluated the program when it was over and ranked exercise as one of the most useful components. In fact, they suggested beefing up the workout sessions and offering even more exercise. Odds are, you'll feel the same way once you start our fitness program.

Best of all, you can do our workout on your own time, in your own house, with little upfront investment. Sounds simple, but an anytime, anywhere routine is what many of us need most. The lack of affordable, accessible fitness programs in the black community often prevents sisters who want to shape up from doing so. They don't have a health club close by, so that becomes yet another excuse. But you don't need a gym to lose weight, as our program proves. All you need is an exercise mat, a sturdy chair, a set of dumbbells, a good pair of walking sneakers, and the desire to get fit. And we know you have that!

Getting Ready to Sweat

Before you begin, set up an appointment with your doctor for a complete physical. You should have his or her okay before starting this, or any, exercise plan. You doctor will help you determine your overall health and fitness level, something you need to know from jumpstreet in order to safely ease into fitness. Once you have your doctor's go-ahead, it's time to get moving.

Since no two women are built alike, sister-trainer Mara Hoskin-Thomas, a certified fitness professional based in San Diego, has developed a workout geared to three different weight categories and body types. After all, a sister who's trying to shed 75 pounds has drastically different needs and abilities than a sister out to drop 15 pounds. No matter where you fall on the spectrum, you *can* reach your goal. So what if it takes you a little longer? You share the same commitment as every other sister reading this page. Think of that common bond as you embark on your journey. Remind your sister circle of the broader community of black women who are walking this path with you. Rely on that connection to see you through.

It's in the Genes

You may have your mother's high cheekbones, your father's deep-set mahogany eyes, and your grandmother's smooth-as-silk complexion. But what about your frame? Whose body type foreshadowed your own? Just as we inherit our eyes, nose, hair, and a host of other defining traits from our kin, so it is with our physiques. Genetics play a key role in determining what our bodies look like.

Yes, we can trim down with exercise and diet, but how easily we gain weight, how muscular we are, the roundness of our hips, the thinness of our legs—these and many more body characteristics are all determined genetically. To truly get the best from your workout, it's important to know which body type you fit. That way, you can home in on different aspects of your build and make the most of the body you were born with. Don't get us wrong—you can't change your body type. However, you can make it look its best. Say you gain weight at the drop of a hat. Sorry girlfriend, but you'll always be that way. That's your body type at work. But knowing so gives you a heads-up to your trouble zone. For you, increased aerobic activity may need to be a key element of your workout in order to combat body fat.

So just where do you fit in? There are three body type classifications: endomorph, mesomorph, and ectomorph.

Endomorphs gain weight easily and typically have a round, curvy, hourglass figure. Their body fat percentage tends to be high.

Mesomorphs are naturally muscular and have a lower percentage of body fat.

Ectomorphs are naturally slender and sinewy. They can eat whatever they want and not gain an ounce.

Many women are a combination of body types, typically mesomorph and endomorph—a combo that exercise physiologists call *meso-endomorphs*. This two-in-one type has the muscles and strength of a mesomorph, but the high body fat of an endomorph.

Chances are, if you're reading this book, you're probably an endomorph, mesomorph, or meso-endomorph. That's why our workout offers easy-to-follow general guidelines targeting those body types. The walking program will help you blast fat quickly and comfortably, while the resistance moves will tone and sculpt your muscles. All you have to do is follow the plan geared to your build. More on that later. Right now, let's talk goals.

How Much Should You Lose?

Remember when we advised you to see your doctor before beginning our program? In addition to giving you the thumbs-up to start a fitness plan, your physician can also help you figure out how much weight you need to lose to improve your health. We know you probably have your own ideas about that, but why "guesstimate"? You may believe you need to shed more pounds than you really do, or you might lowball the amount without realizing it. Keep in mind, you're losing weight to improve your health and prolong your life. Wouldn't you rather be absolutely certain of what your goal-weight range should be when something so important is at stake?

That's right. We said range. No one needs to hit an exact number. Trying to do so will only drive you crazy anyway. We don't want you to become chained to the scale, obsessing over a pound here or two pounds there. Having, say, a ten-pound range, gives you room to maneuver. It's also a healthier—and saner— way to look at weight loss and maintenance, since many of us have a "natural" weight anyway. It's the place where your body feels it's supposed to be. For some sisters that might be anywhere from 135 to 145 pounds; for others it could be 155 to 165, and so on. Dip too far below your set-point and your body will fight back by slowing down your metabolism. We've divided the workout here into three weight-loss categories:

1. Up to 20 pounds
2. 20 to 50 pounds
3. 50 pounds or more

As with the body-type breakdown, the guidelines for the exercise plan include specific instructions for the amount of weight you are trying to lose. All you have to do is find your body type in the guidelines for general tips, then locate your weight-loss category and follow the workout directions for specific exercises, frequency, duration, and repetitions. Don't jump to that section just yet though. We want to make sure you know exactly what you're getting into. Don't worry, no psycho drill-sergeant trainer comes with this workout. We simply want you to understand what the two portions of the workout—aerobic and resistance training—mean, plus give you a breakdown of terminology that will help you successfully navigate your fitness journey.

Making Sense of the Jargon

When most of us think of the word "aerobic," we envision a room full of sweaty, panting women jumping around to blasting music. Well, that's only part of the picture. Aerobic actually means "in the presence of oxygen." When we say aerobic exercise, we mean exercise that requires oxygen. You're engaged in a physical activity that uses your large muscle groups (back, chest, arms, legs, abdominals) so vigorously and intensely—such as jogging, brisk walking, cycling, swimming, or a funk aerobics class—that the muscles need extra energy to keep going. That energy comes from oxygen. Because aerobic exercise feeds a continual supply of oxygen to the muscles, you are able to sustain the activity for a long period of time.

Anaerobic exercise, on the other hand, means exercising "without oxygen." Sounds impossible, but there are exercises that tap energy from sources within the muscles themselves, not from oxygen—for example, strength-training. Because anaerobic exercise fatigues muscles quickly, it can only be sustained for short periods of time.

The walking portion of our workout is the aerobic component;

the resistance moves (also called strength-training) are the anaerobic part. For the best results, you need to do both. Aerobics strengthens your heart and helps you burn fat—especially important for sisters, since we typically have a higher ratio of fat to lean body mass than white women do—while strength-training builds and tones muscle (remember, muscle burns fat too), which in turn revs up your metabolism. Add a series of stretches to the mix and you'll have the most well-rounded, effective workout possible. Gentle, static stretches (no bouncing!) increase your flexibility, help prevent injuries, and give you a leaner, longer look. Now that you've got a handle on aerobic versus anaerobic exercise, familiarize yourself with a few more, equally important terms before you break a sweat.

Repetitions. Abbreviated to "reps," this term refers to the number of times you repeat an exercise. It's typically used in strength-training workouts. For instance, if you're doing bicep curls, and the instructions call for 8 reps, that simply means you are to do 8 bicep curls.

Sets. Also usually a strength-workout term, a "set" is a group of repetitions. Again, imagine you're doing bicep curls. If the workout calls for 2 sets of 8 reps, that means you are to do 8 bicep curls, rest for 30 to 60 seconds, then do another 8 curls.

Resting Heart Rate. This term refers to how fast your heart beats when you're doing nothing. To figure it out, take your pulse while you're resting. Place your fingertips on the radial artery in your inner wrist, straight down from the base of the thumb. Count the beats for ten seconds. Multiply that number by six. The result is your estimated resting heart rate. Do this for three mornings in a row; add up the numbers and divide the sum by three to get an average. You can also take your pulse at your neck. Place your index and middle fingers by the outside corner of one eye and slide them straight down to the carotid artery in your neck. Be sure not to press your free hand against the other side of your neck at the same time, because doing so could impede blood flow, rendering your heart-rate measurement inaccurate. Don't use your thumb, either, because it has its own pulse.

Target Heart Rate. This refers to the maximum rate at which your heart can pump safely during aerobic exercise. To get the most from your workout, and strengthen your heart and lungs, you should aim to work within your target heart-rate range, typically 60 to 80 percent of your maximum heart rate. To calculate your target heart rate, subtract your age from 220, then multiple that number by .6 and .8. The result is your target heart rate. So if you are forty years old, your maximum heart rate is 180 and your target heart range is 108 to 144. This is your "zone." You want to work within it to get the best results. Keep track of your heart rate (pulse) as you work out, and if you're new to exercise, stay at the lower end of your zone—so in the example above, you wouldn't allow your heart rate to go higher than 125. If it does, slow down your workout a bit because you're pushing too hard. As you move from a novice to a more intermediate and advanced exerciser, you can strive to work at the higher end of your zone.

Target Heart Rate At-a-Glance

AGE	60%	80%
20	120	160
25	117	156
30	114	152
35	111	148
40	108	144
45	105	140
50	102	136
55	99	132
60	96	128

The *Slim Down Sister* Workout

Body-Type Guidelines

Endomorph. Since you gain weight easily, you need to keep your aerobic work at a higher level than your resistance work. This way you'll keep body fat under control while still boosting your lean muscle mass.

Mesomorph. You tend to gain muscle quickly, so you'd do well to use light weights and high reps in your strength-training to avoid packing on more bulk. Just because you have a lower percentage of body fat, though, doesn't mean you can skip the cardio. Strive for a balance between your aerobic work and your resistance work.

Meso-Endomorph. You've got the best of both worlds. That's right, the *best*. Think about it, girl. You have the sexy curves of a mesomorph and the strength of an endomorph. To burn off that top layer of fat and get to the muscles underneath, you should go for the same revved up aerobic work as a mesomorph and the moderate strength-training of an endomorph.

Weight-Loss Category Guidelines

Up to 20 pounds. Do the walking program three to four days a week and do your specific resistance moves two to three days a week.

20 to 50 pounds. Walk four to five days a week and do your specific resistance exercises three days a week.

50 pounds or more. Walk five days a week and do your specific resistance moves three days a week.

Walk Off the Weight

Walking is one of the easiest ways to shed pounds. Not only does it burn fat fast and effectively, it also improves your cardiovascular health, lowers blood pressure and blood cholesterol, increases bone strength, and puts you at low risk for injury. A few things to keep in mind before you lace up your sneakers: Map out your route ahead of time and let a family member or friend know where you'll be. Make sure your walking route is safe and free of obstructions. If you will be walking near traffic early in the morning or in the evening, wear brightly colored clothing and reflective strips so drivers can see you. Take a bottle of water with you to stay hydrated. Before you hit your stride, make sure to warm up by walking a bit slower than exercise pace for five or ten minutes. When your workout is done, cool down by walking slowly for another five or ten minutes, and finish up with a few easy stretches—hold each one for 30 seconds with no bouncing.

You have to use good form when you walk to truly reap the fitness benefits. Here's how to put your best foot forward: Keep your chest lifted and your eyes focused ahead. Use proper heel-to-toe technique—land on your heel, roll the entire length of your foot on the ground, and push off with your toes. Keep your abdominals slightly contracted. Breathe deeply as you walk—in through the nose, out through the mouth. Swing arms naturally at your sides to start; as you build up speed, begin pumping your arms at a 90-degree angle to help propel yourself forward. Test your intensity by seeing how well you can talk while walking. You're working in the proper zone if you're breathing hard but are still able to carry on a conversation. If you're so out of breath that you can't talk, that means you're pushing too hard.

You may want to buy a pedometer to keep track of how many miles you're covering. These inexpensive little gadgets, available at sporting goods stores, clip right onto your clothes and tally distance, time, and steps. Or you can simply jump in your car ahead of time and use the odometer to figure out how far it is from your house to various places in your neighborhood. Then as you walk from place to place, you'll know how far you've gone. Either way, the point is to determine your progress from week to week. When you first begin, it may take you 30 or 35 minutes to walk one mile. You want to whittle that time down until you can do a 15-minute mile consistently. Keep at it and you'll be there before you know it.

For now, though, start off slowly and at a comfortable pace. Don't worry about how fast you're going just yet. At this point, you're simply trying to ease your way into it. Your first goal is to walk for 20 minutes. Build up to it if you have to, going a little longer every day until you're up to 20 consistent minutes. Pick up the pace from week to week. Try to go a little faster each time you walk, but always maintain good form. Then move up to 30 minutes, increasing speed incrementally as you go. Keep in mind that your goal is to lose weight and improve your health, and a stroll just won't cut it. Easy walking is fine in the first week or two, but remember, you have to make the effort to walk more quickly each time you head out the door. Putting pep in your step is the key to shaving off inches and pounds. Once you're at half-hour walks, nudge it up to 45 minutes. Break your walks into 15-minute shots if you have to, say in the morning, at lunch, and after dinner. How you break things up doesn't matter, as long as you work them in.

When you can do 45 minute walks at a 15-minute-per-mile pace, give yourself a pat on the back. This translates to three miles for every outing. You go, girl! Want to kick it up to an hour? Be our guest. Just make sure to test yourself slowly and easily. Try too much too soon and your body will definitely let you know about it. Heed your body's messages.

Get Pumped

Why pump iron? Because it works those muscles, sisterfriend. The more you have, the more efficiently your body can burn calories. In fact, one pound of muscle burns 35 calories a day. Plus you'll increase your strength levels, stave off osteoporsis by building denser bones, and give your body a leaner, sleeker look.

You don't have to lift weights to "pump," however. Your own body offers plenty of resistance. The idea is to work against some type of resistance, be it from a dumbbell or from your own body weight. Our program is a combination of both. And since sisters tend to carry excess weight in the waist-to-hip area, we've made sure to include midsection moves that really work those abs. Don't worry, you're not going to end up looking like Ah-nuld. Using light to moderate resistance won't turn you into a female bodybuilder—you'd have to hoist some seriously heavy weights for that. What this routine will do is carve out sleek, sexy curves. You'll look toned and tight, not big and bulky. Ready to give it a go? You'll need an exercise mat, a sturdy chair, and a pair of 2- to 3-pound dumbbells to start (as you progress, increase to 5-pound, then 8-pound weights). Now simply find your weight-loss category and follow the instructions—be sure to warm up by marching in place for a few minutes before starting. Whichever weight-loss category you fit, do the first program for six weeks, then move to program #2 for six weeks, then it's on to program #3 for six weeks. Instructions for doing each exercise are given beginning on page 61.

You don't want to feel restricted when you work out, so make sure to wear clothes that are comfortable and nonbinding. But make sure they aren't too loose and flowing or they may get in the way as you exercise. Continue rotating every six weeks to keep boredom and plateaus at bay. As you do these exercises, pay attention to your breathing. Exhale on the action, and inhale on the release. Remember, too, that slower is better. Let your muscles, not momentum, do the work.

Up to 20 pounds—Program #1

Lunge—Do 3 sets of 15 reps
Upright Row—Do 3 sets of 12 reps
Push-Up—Do 2 sets of 10 reps
Reverse Crunch—Do 3 sets of 15 reps

Up to 20 pounds—Program #2

Squat—Do 3 sets of 15 reps
Bicep Curl—Do 3 sets of 10 reps
Anterior Raise—Do 3 sets of 10 reps
Basic Crunch—Do 3 sets of 15 reps

Up to 20 pounds—Program #3

Tricep Kickback—Do 3 sets of 10 reps
Plié Squat—Do 3 sets of 10 reps
Basic Crunch—Do 2 sets of 15 reps
Oblique Twist—Do 3 sets of 15 reps

20 to 50 pounds—Program #1

Lunge—Do 3 sets of 8 reps
Bicep Curl—Do 2 sets of 10 reps
Lateral Raise—Do 2 sets of 10 reps
Basic Crunch—Do 2 sets of 15 reps

20 to 50 pounds—Program #2

Squat—Do 3 sets of 15 reps
Tricep Kickback—Do 2 sets of 10 reps
Chair Push-Up—Do 2 sets of 12 reps
Oblique Twist—Do 2 sets of 15 reps

20 to 50 pounds—Program #3

Plié Squat—Do 3 sets of 12 reps
Military Press—Do 2 sets of 12 reps
One-Arm Row—Do 2 sets of 12 reps
Basic Crunch—Do 2 sets of 15 reps

50 pounds or more—Program #1

Lunge—Do 3 sets of 8 reps
Plié Squat—Do 3 sets of 10 reps

Chair Push-Up—Do 2 sets of 10 reps
Basic Crunch—Do 2 sets of 15 reps

50 pounds or more—Program #2

Hamstring Curl—Do 3 sets of 15 reps
Tricep Kickback—Do 2 sets of 10 reps
Oblique Twist—Do 2 sets of 15 reps
Chair Squat—Do 3 sets of 15 reps

50 pounds or more—Program #3

Squat—Do 3 sets of 15 reps
Calf Raise—Do 3 sets of 15 reps
Bicep Curl—Do 3 sets of 10 reps
Basic Crunch—Do 2 sets of 15 reps

How to Do the Moves

Anterior Raise

1. Stand with feet hip-width apart, knees slightly bent, and abs contracted. Hold one weight in each hand at your sides.

2. With elbows slightly bent, slowly lift your arms in front of you up to shoulder level. Don't go higher than shoulder height. Slowly bring your arms back down to your sides. Repeat.

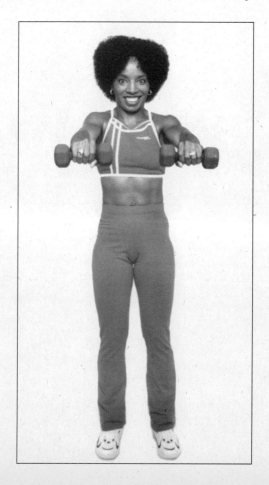

Basic Crunch

1. Lie on your back with knees bent and feet flat on floor. Hands should be behind your head (but don't lace your fingers), elbows out to the sides. Contract your abdominal muscles.

2. Slowly curl up until your shoulder-blades are off the ground. Keep your eyes focused on the ceiling to keep your chin from resting on your chest. Lower back down to the starting position. Repeat.

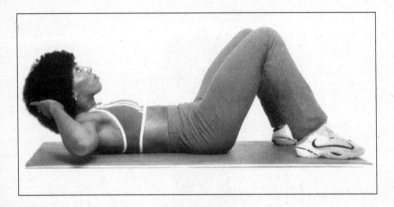

Bicep Curl

1. Stand with feet hip-width apart, knees slightly bent, abs in, and holding weights at your sides, palms facing forward.

2. Keeping elbows close to your waist, lift weights up toward your shoulders. Lower slowly back to the starting position. Repeat.

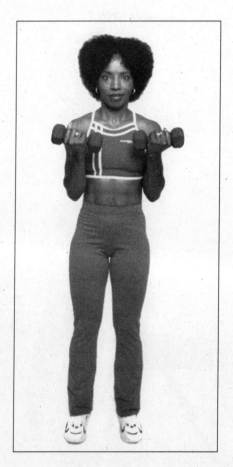

Calf Raise

1. Place your hands on a chair for support. With your feet close together, press up onto your toes.

2. Slowly press your heels toward the floor without actually touching the floor. Then lift back up onto your toes. Repeat.

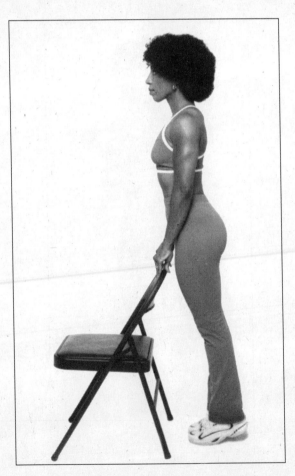

Hamstring Curl

1. Stand with feet hip-width apart. Hold on to a chair for support. Extend your left leg behind you.

2. Bend your left knee and flex your left foot, bringing your left heel toward your buttocks. Make sure to squeeze. Return to start position. Complete reps and repeat with opposite leg.

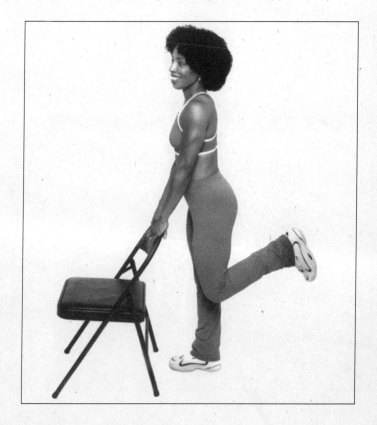

Lateral Raise

1. Stand with feet hip-width apart, abs in, knees slightly bent. Hold weights at your sides with your palms facing in.

2. With elbows slightly bent, slowly lift arms out to the sides and up to shoulder level (don't go higher than that) with palms facing down. Slowly lower arms, leading with your wrists. Repeat.

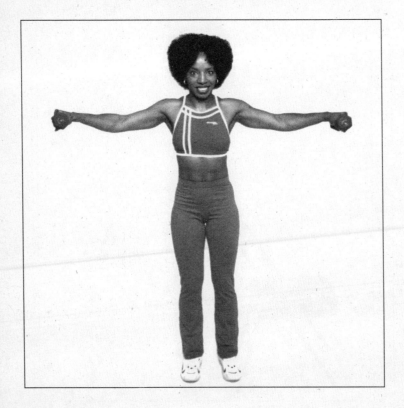

Lunge

1. Stand with feet hip-width apart and abs in. Rest hands on hips. Step right leg forward about three feet.

2. Slowly lower torso until both knees make 90 degree angles. Be sure your left knee does not go lower than ankle level. Don't lean forward. Lift back up to start position. Complete reps and repeat with opposite leg.

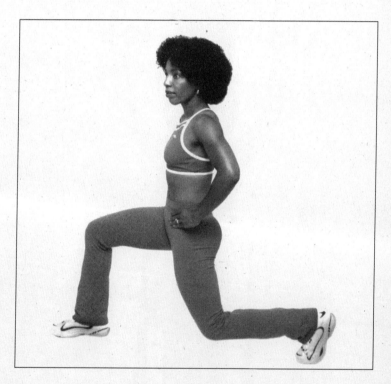

Military Press

1. Sit in a chair with feet flat on the floor, back straight, abs in. With a weight in each hand, raise hands to shoulders, palms facing forward. Elbows should point straight down.

2. Slowly extend your arms up (without locking your elbows), then slowly lower back down to shoulder level. Repeat.

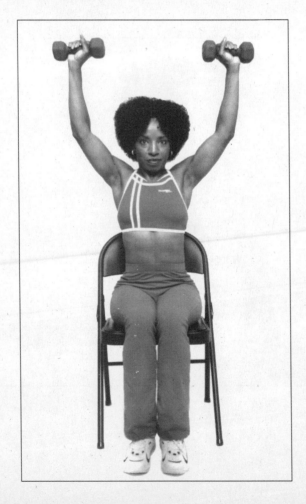

Oblique Twist

1. Lie on your back with knees bent and feet flat on the floor. Place hands behind head (don't lace fingers), elbows out to sides.

2. Slowly curl up, then turn torso slightly to the right. Keep lower back pressed into the floor and try not to tilt your hips and pelvis. Bring torso back to the center, then lower. Repeat on the left side.

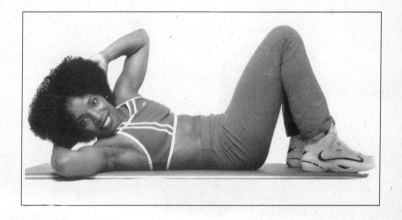

One-Arm Row

1. Stand with your right foot forward and knee bent. Lean forward and place your right hand on right thigh. Head, back, and left leg should be in line. Hold a dumbbell in your left hand and extend it to the floor, with your palm facing in.

2. Keeping your back flat, bend your left elbow and slowly bring the weight up to your torso. Lower back to start position. Repeat.

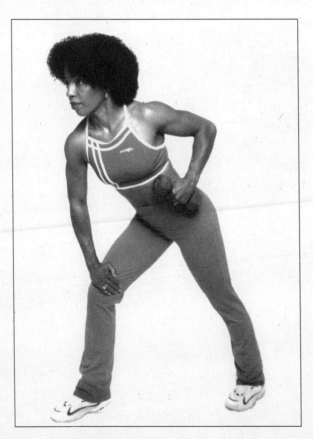

Plié Squat

1. Stand with your feet several inches past hip-width apart, toes and knees facing out. Place hands on hips and contract abs.

2. Bend knees and lower torso. Do not lean forward. Push down on your heels and lift back up. Repeat.

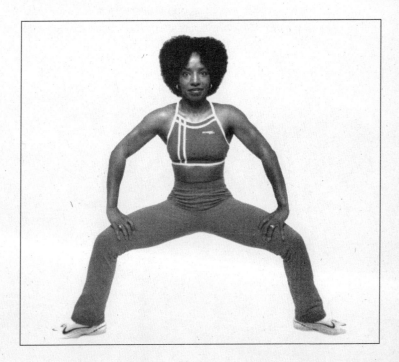

Push-Up

1. Get down on hands and knees with arms extended and hands slightly more than shoulder-width apart, fingers pointing forward. Lift feet and cross ankles; pull abs in. Body should be in a straight diagonal line from knees to head.

2. Bend elbows, slowly lowering body until upper arms are parallel to the floor. Keep your abs contracted. Push back up. Repeat.

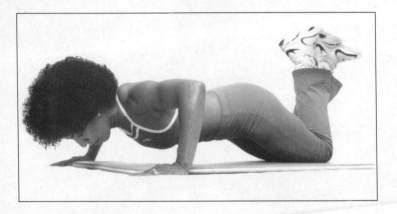

Reverse Crunch

1. Lie on your back with legs up and slightly bent. Feet are together. (If this position is too difficult, bend knees to a 45-degree angle.) Cross arms over your chest.

2. Tighten your abs and lift hips a bit off the ground. Hold for a second, then lower. Focus on lifting with the lower part of your abdominal muscles, not your hip muscles. Repeat.

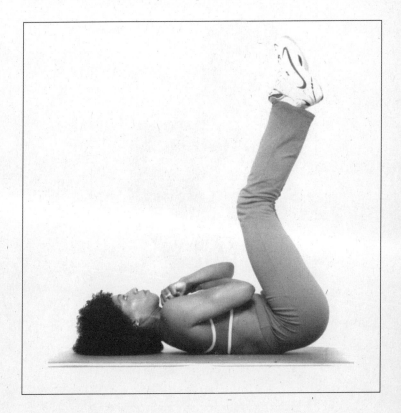

Squat

1. Stand with feet a few inches apart and abs contracted. Rest hands on hips.

2. Bend knees and sit back as if to sit in a chair. Do not let hips go lower than your knees. Press down on your heels and lift back up to start position. Repeat.

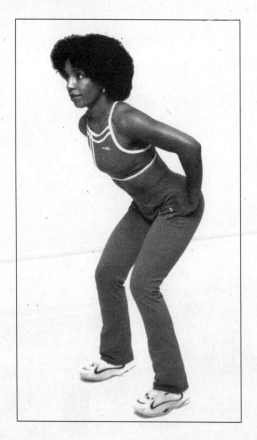

Tricep Kickback

1. Stand with your right foot forward and right knee bent. Lean forward and place your right hand on right thigh. Head, back, and left leg should be in line. Hold a dumbbell in your left hand and extend it to the floor, with your palm facing in. Keeping your back flat, bend your left elbow and bring the weight up to your torso.

2. Extend your left forearm back behind you. Return to start position. Repeat.

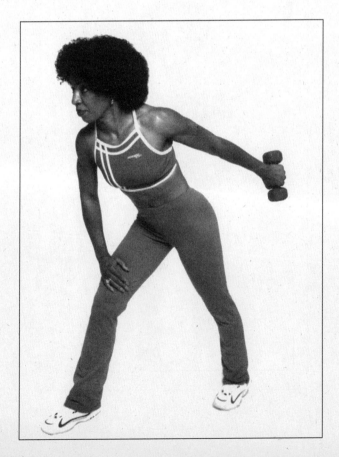

Upright Row

1. Stand with feet hip-width apart, knees slightly bent, abs contracted. Hold a dumbbell in each hand close together in front of your thighs. Your palms should be facing your thighs.

2. Bend your elbows and lift the weights up to chest level. (Try to work up to collarbone level, with elbows slightly above shoulder height.) Lower back to start position. Repeat.

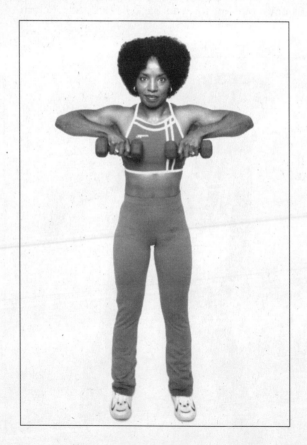

Chair Push-Up

1. Stand arm's length from a chair, with hands on the chair about shoulder-width apart. Elbows should be slightly bent, and abdominal muscles contracted.

2. Bend your elbows and lean in toward the chair, keeping your abs in and your back straight. Push off the chair back to start position. Repeat.

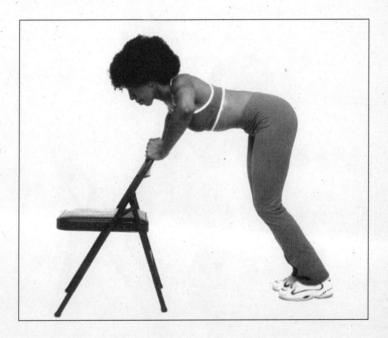

Chair Squat

1. Stand about two feet in front of a chair with your feet a few inches apart, toes pointing forward. Clasp your hands together in front of your thighs.

2. Slowly bend your knees and lower your torso until your buttocks lightly touch the chair. As you lower your torso, bring your arms up in front of you to chest level, keeping your hands clasped. Slowly lift up. Repeat.

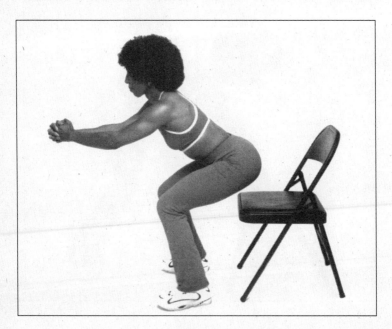

Sister to Sister
XOXOXOXOX

Rosalyn Bower Harrison, a thirty-seven-year-old certified registered nurse anesthetist from Detroit, Michigan
Current weight: 160 pounds
Amount lost: 35 pounds

I know exactly why I put on weight: marriage and school. After I got married I was comfortable and in a relaxed environment. I wasn't out there living that single life, putting on the fancy clothes, going to the clubs, you know what I mean. I was settled and I was gaining weight.

I was also in school, and all I did was go to school, study, go to school, study. It was very stressful, so I ate. And I put on more weight.

I didn't pass my anesthesia boards the first time I took them, and that made me very depressed. What did I do? Eat, eat, and eat. And I put on even more weight.

In my profession, the only thing we wear in the hospital is scrubs. So it wasn't like I had to put on nice clothes to go to work. When I got home from the hospital, I'd put on a jogging suit or something like that. All the clothes I wore were pretty loose-fitting. I knew I'd gained weight, but I couldn't really see it, you know?

When I looked at myself in the mirror I didn't see anything different. I just saw the same person. I figured I'd put on 5 or 10 pounds here or there, nothing major. I didn't realize how much it actually was until I got on the scale.

It was a comment from my girlfriend that made me step on the scale. I ran into her one day and she said, "Oh, Ros, you've gained so much weight. What is wrong with you?" What really got me is that my friend made that comment in front of a lot of people. It was so embarrassing. After that incident I felt that people were looking at me and thinking that I'd gained a lot. What's worse, my husband talked about my weight all the time, telling me I was getting too big. He made negative comments constantly and it irritated the heck out of me.

When I finally stepped on the scale and it read 195, I almost had a fit. I felt depressed and uncomfortable with myself. I didn't want to go anywhere. Luckily, I didn't have high blood pressure or any other health problems. And I sure didn't want any to crop up. So I started working out and eating better.

I read several magazine articles about nutrition and healthy eating and used the information to create my own eating plan. I stopped eating fried food and sweets, except for twice a month. I ate chicken and fish at least three times a week. I also had a lot of pasta and vegetables. I went out to dinner twice a month and allowed myself to eat whatever I wanted. That's when I'd have the fried food and dessert.

I exercised faithfully, too. I did aerobic tapes at home three or four times a week, and walked in a park near my home on the other days (one time around the park equaled three miles). All told, I was exercising five to six days a week for about 45 minutes each time.

I put pictures of Janet Jackson and Oprah on my refrigerator for inspiration. My belly button kept me motivated too. I had it pierced awhile back and I always said that I was going to show off my belly-button ring someday.

I wasn't always perfect. When I had cravings, I'd sometimes indulge, but never to the point where I was thrown off-track. I knew losing weight was something I had to do. Since I'm in the health profession, I see a number of overweight sisters with high blood pressure and other problems. I knew I'd benefit more in the long run if I got fit. So I kept thinking about that every day.

As I lost weight, I felt better about my health and became very proud of myself. I felt good, girl. Ten months after I started, I had lost 45 pounds. I've put ten back on because my life became very stressful again. I separated from my husband and moved back in with my parents for a while until I could find a place of my own. I was in transition and I was depressed about my situation. When I'm depressed I eat. But I'm back on track now. I have my own place, I recently joined an aerobics class at a local recreation center, and I'm refocused on eating right. I'm definitely going to nip this minor regain in the bud. I have confidence in myself and I no longer worry about what other people say. Some folks give off such negative energy. You just have to ignore it and set your mind to what you want to do.

Remember what I said about my belly-button ring? Well, I went to Aruba on vacation this year and I wore a two-piece bathing suit. Girl, you know I was showing off my belly button.

CHAPTER 5

⊗

Let's Eat!
Keeping the Flava,
Losing the Fat

B lack folks love good food. Think about those big family dinners you share with kin. The food is always spread out on the
dining room table like a feast. Ham, macaroni and cheese, collards,
ribs, potato salad, snap beans, fried chicken, banana pudding—
the works. It may be Kwanzaa or Christmas, Sunday supper after
services, or just an impromptu get-together. Whatever the occasion,
our people celebrate with a bounty of nourishment. Even when
the setting is more intimate or everyday—say, dinner for two or a
meal with the kids—flavors of our past lovingly fill each dish.

Through the generations, the culinary skills and techniques
that our great-great-grandmothers passed on to their daughters
have been passed down to us. Pot liquor isn't a "waste," it's an essential. Ox tails aren't something to be discarded; they're a food
to be relished. The way we prepare our meals is second nature.
Many of us don't even have to think about it. We just head on
into the kitchen and get to cooking. We know instinctively what's
needed to give our favorite foods that "flava." The right combination of ingredients can make or break soulful cuisine. So we stick
to tradition. If that's the way Mama made it, that's the way we're
going to make it too.

The Food of Survival

What drives our strong feelings about what we eat and the way we cook? History. Soul food is the food of survivors. The legacy is in our blood; it's an inherent part of who we are as a people. We may not consciously think of our ancestry as we lovingly prepare soul food dishes whose recipes have been orally handed down for years, but somewhere inside us, we recognize the significance of those favorite meals. Our forefathers' West African roots are clearly evident in many of the foods we eat today—okra, yams, black-eyed peas, corn, rice. And their struggle to survive slavery deeply influences our food preferences and cooking methods.

As slaves, our people had to make do with scraps from the master's table. Even though they were forced to eat the lesser, fattier parts of the pig—the intestines (chitlins), the stomach, the neck, and the hocks—along with other leftover rations, our ancestors managed to supplement their diet by hunting and fishing, and by cultivating vegetables in small gardens. From these scraps, fish, game, and home-grown vegetables, they created rich, flavorful, imaginative dishes reflective of their African culinary traditions, such as stews and one-pot meals—staples of our current cuisine. Over time, the foods and cooking methods of our ancestors' origins melded with those of the American South, evolving into the modern form of soul food that we enjoy today.

Fortunately, many of the foods we love are rich in nutrients. Okra and collards, for instance, are high in vitamin C. Yams and sweet potatoes are bursting with vitamin A. Dry beans offer a wealth of protein. Other favorites, like catfish, corn, shrimp, and cruciferous vegetables (cabbage, greens, and the like) are chock-full of cancer-fighting nutrients. It's simply the way we prepare them that compromises their healthfulness. Take greens. What soul food menu would be complete without greens like collards, kale, spinach, and turnip greens, just to name a few. Each has a wonderful and distinctive taste that fills the senses with memories of the South. Each is also high in beta-carotene, vitamin C, and fiber. But because we boil greens with salt pork, fatback, or hamhocks, we pump up the fat and salt content while stripping away some of the vital nutrients.

Time for a Change

The good news is, to lose weight and improve our health, we don't have to give up the down-home tastes we savor. Nor should we. Soul food is too important a part of black cultural identity. What we *can* do, however, is resolve to prepare these treasured dishes more healthfully. Not only will we shed pounds, we'll also improve upon the culinary traditions that will one day be passed on to our own children.

Deep down, most sisters know it's time for a change. Scores of you have told us as much. We hold health fairs for black women all over the country, and time and time again sisters ask us what they should be eating in order to get fit. The fact that thousands of black women just like you attend these fairs proves to us that sisters want to better their health, lengthen their lives, and find a feasible way to take off excess weight. But when it comes to food, they simply aren't sure what to do. Here's the main complaint we've heard from you over the years: "No one has explained to me how to eat healthfully without giving up the foods I love." In fact, over a third of African-Americans cite giving up foods as the most common barrier to achieving a nutritious eating style, according to a 1997 American Dietetic Association survey of nutrition trends. That really is the bottom line: When sisters seek advice from experts, they're given nutritional information that simply doesn't speak to them. You don't see any of the soulful foods you enjoy every day on those meal plans, so of course you believe that there's no room for soul food in a smart eating program. Well, we're here to tell you there is. The trick is to relegate those foods to their proper place—and the Soul Food Pyramid can show you how.

A Pyramid with Soul

Based on the USDA Food Guide Pyramid, which classifies the six major food groups and offers servings guidelines for a well-balanced, healthy diet, the Soul Food Pyramid takes it a step further. The traditional pyramid, while providing sound guidelines, never addresses the particular food preferences of African-Americans. And if sisters are to adopt healthier ways of eating, they can't be expected to do it by giving up foods they love. That's a surefire formula for failure. Sooner or later you'll feel deprived. Once that happens, it's just a matter of time before you say, "Forget this," and resume old eating habits.

What we've done is keep those down-home favorites on the menu—bet you won't find chitlins and grits on the traditional pyramid—but in their proper place. You simply have to start viewing soul food in a different way in order to keep eating it and still lose weight. Think neckbones with collards, sweet potatoes, and cornbread make a meal? Think again. Let's just take one part of that dinner—neckbones. We're not telling you to stop eating them altogether. What we are saying is really think about what they are: A fat to be eaten on occasion, not a meat to be consumed twice a week. For generations, black folks have been eating these sorts of meats as if they were like any other meat. But they're not. Their fat content is so high that they must be considered fats.

See the problem? We tend to use fatty meats as the protein base of many dinners. But you can't treat neckbones like chicken or fish. You have to let go of that mind-set if you're going to bolster your health.

The Soul Food Pyramid shows you—literally (check out the pictures)—how to categorize neckbones and other high-fat meats.

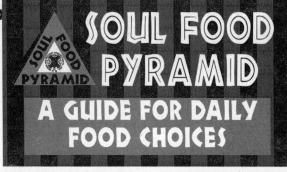

SOUL FOOD PYRAMID

A GUIDE FOR DAILY FOOD CHOICES

The Soul Food Pyramid emphasizes foods from all major food groups of the Pyramid. These food groups provide some, but not all, of the nutrients you need for a healthy diet. The foods in one group cannot replace those in another. The foods in all groups are equally important for good health.

The Pyramid is an outline of what you should eat each day. This is only a general guide that will assist you in choosing a healthy diet that is right for you. The Pyramid calls for eating a variety of foods to get the nutrients you need and to get the right amount of calories needed to maintain a healthy weight.

Fats, Oils & Sweets
(eat sparingly)

Milk, Cheese
& Yogurt Group
2–3 Servings

Fruit Group
2–4 Servings

Meats, Poultry, Fish, Dry
Beans, Eggs & Nuts Group
2–3 Servings

Vegetables Group
3–5 Servings

Breads, Cereal,
Rice & Pasta Group
6–11 Servings

FOOD GROUPS	GRAPHIC OF FOOD GROUPS	ONE SERVING EQUALS ONE ITEM	CALORIES		
			1,600 Many Women and Older Adults	2,200 Children, Teen Girls, Active Women, and Most Men	2,800 Teen Boys and Active Men
Eat Liberally 6–11 servings daily Breads, Cereal, Rice & Pasta Group		1 slice white or brown bread ½ hamburger bun 1 biscuit (1–2" diameter) ½ cup rice, grits, macaroni, or noodles 1 cup ready-to-eat cereal (flake/nonsugar-coated) ½ cup cooked cereal (oatmeal or cream of wheat) 2–4 crackers ½ bagel	6	9	11
Eat Generously 3–5 servings daily Vegetables Group		1 cup raw, green leafy vegetables ½ cup cooked vegetable (collards, okra, snap beans, pole beans, turnips, kale, mustard greens, green cabbage, potatoes, sweet potatoes, squash, corn, carrots, and onions) ¾ cup low-sodium vegetable juice	3	4	5
Eat Generously 2–4 servings daily Fruit Group		Eat a variety of fruits, such as medium apple, banana, peach, mango, orange, pear, ½ grapefruit, ¼ cantaloupe, ½ cup grapes, 1 cup of strawberries or blackberries ¾ cup 100% fruit juice (not fruit punch or presweetened drink) ½ cup canned fruit packed in light syrup or fruit (natural) juice	2	3	4
Eat Moderately 2–3 servings daily Meats, Poultry, Fish, Dry Beans, Eggs & Nuts Group		2 servings for females, 6 oz total daily 3 servings for males, 7 oz total daily 3 oz poultry, lean beef, fish, lean pork Eggs (3 per week) 3 oz lean lamb or lean ground meats ½ cup cooked or dried peas or beans 1 tablespoon of peanut butter (limit servings) ¼ cup nuts Note: Bake, broil, grill, stew, or boil meats whenever possible. Limit use of shellfish due to high cholesterol content.	2	2–3	3
Eat Moderately 2–3 servings daily Milk, Cheese & Yogurt Group		1 cup milk or buttermilk (1% or skim milk recommended) 1 cup lactose-free milk ½ cup ice cream, ice milk, or low-fat frozen yogurt 1 ½ oz natural cheese (cheddar, colby, provolone, mozzarella) ½ cup cottage cheese 1 cup low-fat yogurt	2	2–3	3
Eat Sparingly Snacks & Sweets Group		Snacks, sweets, cakes, pies, cookies, and other desserts: Eat in moderation, go easy on rich desserts, candies, soft drinks, and alcoholic beverages. Snack-foods items, such as chips, cheese puffs, corn chips, and pork skins should be eaten only occasionally because they are high in sugar, fat, and salt. These foods do not have enough nutrients to fit in any of the basic food groups and should not be used to replace foods from other food groups.			
Eat Sparingly Fats, Oils & Sweets Group		The small tip of the Pyramid shows high-fat meats, snacks, vegetable fats and oils, salt, and sweets. Foods such as chitterlings, sausage, bacon, pork neckbones, fat back, hog jowls, and pigs feet are traditionally used in the African-American diet as meats. Due to the high fat content, these foods belong to the Fats, Oils & Sweets Group and should be used sparingly. Foods in this group provide calories that are low in nutri-ents. Vegetable oils contain essential fatty acids, but use these sparingly because they are high in calories. For every tablespoon of fat added to 2,200-calorie diet, you increase the percentage of calories as fat by approximately 5 percent (110 calories).			

*Use visible fats sparingly.
*Limit desserts to two or three per week, with regular meal.
*Use honey, jams, jelly, corn syrups, molasses, sugar sparingly.
*Use soft drinks and candies very sparingly, if at all.
*Limit foods high in salt.
*Avoid lard.

1 gm fat = 9 calories

1 tsp salt (table salt) = 2,000 mg sodium
1 tsp oil = 40.0 calories, 4.5 g fat
1 tsp margarine = 34 calories, 3.8 g fat
1 tsp butter = 34 calories, 3.8 g fat
1 tbsp mayonnaise = 100 calories, 10 g fat

1 tbsp sour cream = 31 calories, 3.0 g fat
1 tbsp cream cheese = 49 calories, 4.9 g fat
1 tbsp cream = 51 calories, 5.5 g fat
1 tsp sugar = 16 calories
3 oz chitterlings = 258 calories, 24 g fat

That's not all. You'll find everything from biscuits and grits to okra and sweet potatoes on the pyramid. Sisters' food preferences are definitely represented here. We want you to be satisfied as you lose weight. No matter how soulful your tastes, you'll be able to make your meals healthful with our guidelines.

Figuring Out Food Groups

A quick scan of your kitchen will likely reveal too many processed foods and too few fruits and vegetables. Black folks' diets are sorely lacking in these nutritious foods. If there's one thing you should keep in mind, it's that a well-rounded diet that balances calories with nutrients is essential to lose weight the right way. In a nutshell, you need variety, balance, and moderation. To get all three, you have to eat from the major food groups. Do so, and you should have no problem making your taste buds dance.

The Soul Food Pyramid is divided into six food groups:

Breads, cereals, rice, and pasta (6 to 11 servings a day). This group is the foundation of the pyramid, and includes such favorites as grits, biscuits, and macaroni. All of the foods in this group are made from grains and are excellent sources of complex carbohydrates. What's so important about that? Well, complex carbs give us the energy and fuel we need to keep going every day. Grains and cereals—especially those that are enriched—also supply us with B vitamins (thiamin, niacin, riboflavin), iron, and folic acid. Another plus: Grain-based foods contain very little fat or cholesterol—a good thing, to be sure. But we do run into problems when we eat processed foods in this group, such as croissants, pastries, donuts, crackers, and other refined breads. These items tend to be high in fat because of the way they are prepared.

Vegetables (3 to 5 servings a day). Sisters need to add more veggies to their diet. In fact, you'd do well to consume the high end of the serving recommendation—5 servings a day. Trust us, you'll be doing your health a favor, because deep yellow vegetables and dark leafy greens are excellent sources of beta-carotene, vitamin A, and a host of other nutrients. Fortunately, many soul food staples, including collards, kale, and sweet potatoes, fit the bill. Vegetables also provide us with fiber.

Fruit (2 to 4 servings a day). As with vegetables, fruits are not well represented in sisters' diets either. And they should be. Fruits are fat- and cholesterol-free, and are excellent sources of vitamin C, especially citrus fruits such as oranges. Deep yellow fruits—like mangoes, cantaloupe, peaches—are high in vitamin A. Bananas are great for potassium. For extra nutrients, leave the peel on apples, peaches, and pears.

Meats, poultry, fish, dry beans, eggs, and nuts (2 to 3 servings a day). Black folks tend to consume an excess of foods from this group, especially meat. While we need protein in our diet, it's important that we maintain variety and keep an eye on portion size. Meats are good sources of iron, zinc, and B vitamins (thiamin, niacin, B_6 and B_{12}), however, make sure to select lean cuts, and always trim off excess fat. This is particularly important for us, since we tend to favor high-fat meats. If you typically eat inexpensive ground beef, you might be surprised to learn that 4 ounces of it can contain as much as 37 grams of fat. Compare that to lean ground sirloin: 4 ounces has only 8 grams of fat. Fish, skinless poultry, lean beef, or legumes should be consumed daily, but make them only one-fourth of the servings on your plate.

Milk, cheese, and yogurt (2 to 3 servings a day). These foods are chock-full of vitamin D, calcium, and riboflavin. Milk, in particular, is an excellent source of protein, phosphorus, potassium, and vitamins A and D. Keep in mind that the dairy group can be high in fat and cholesterol, though the amounts will vary by product. That's why it makes sense to opt for low-fat choices, such as skim and one-percent milk. If you are one of the many African-Americans who are lactose-intolerant, try low-fat, lactose-free milk.

Fats, oils, and sweets (eat sparingly). You'll see that on the Soul Food Pyramid, meats such as chitlins, neckbones, pigs' feet, and the like have been added to this food group. That's because they are high in fat, and like sweets and oils should not be eaten too often. Sisters love this food group because it contains items that help lend our favorite foods that certain flavor. You don't have to forgo the foods here, but moderation is required. In addition to being high in fat, these foods are also packed with calories that are low in nutrients.

Consider the six food groups, then consider the foods you usually eat. What did you have for breakfast today? How about lunch? Dinner? Did you have any snacks? How does your daily diet stack up? If you didn't do so well, you're not alone. In today's fast-paced world, sisters have a lot going on and it all adds up to no time. It's little wonder sisters want meals that are quick and easy. And when you do have time to cook a hot, hearty meal, you want to indulge. You want to taste the soulful flavors of your mother's and grandmother's kitchen. Between quick-and-easy and down-home, sisters are giving their health short shrift. When you lack time, you probably stick to foods that are convenient and that require little preparation. The problem is that those quick, easy, processed foods are often high in fat, salt, and sugar. On the flip side, when a sister ties on her apron for some fierce cooking, tradition dictates methods that also leave her meals high in fat, salt, and sugar.

So just what are the problems with our typical soul food fare? Selecting cuts of meats and other foods that are high in fat, using smoked meat products that are high in sodium, frying foods, eating too few fruits and vegetables, and not paying enough attention to portion control.

As we've mentioned before, there's a lot of good to be found in our favorite foods. Kale, turnip greens, collards, mustard greens, broccoli, and spinach are high in vitamins A and C. Sweet potatoes, carrots, plantains, yams, acorn squash, and butternut squash offer up lots of vitamin A as well. Various vitamins and minerals, including niacin, B6, zinc, and potassium can be found in green peas, lima beans, corn, potatoes, and rutabaga. And legumes such as black beans, pinto beans, black-eyed peas, lima beans, and navy beans are excellent sources of fiber, protein, thiamin, folate, iron, magnesium, phosphorus, zinc, and potassium.

While we're ticking off everything that's right with our cuisine, let's not forget our Caribbean influences. A sizable Caribbean subculture exists within the black community, so it's not surprising that spicy island dishes and flavors are an integral part of many sisters' menus. Can't you just taste that jerk chicken now? Because it includes a variety of fish, legumes, fruits, rice, and vegetables, the Caribbean diet is healthy at its base. But fans of the food must be careful of sodium. The salted meats widely used in Caribbean recipes up the sodium content.

Shopping with Soul

To change the way you eat, you have to start at the source—the supermarket. When you roll your shopping cart through the door, which aisle do you hit first? Cereal, meats, soda, produce? Are you working from a list or do you buy on the fly? In talking to thousands of black women across the country, we've found that most sisters have pretty erratic shopping patterns. We tend not to use a list, nor do we plan our meals ahead of time so that we'll have some idea of what we truly need. The result? Meals that aren't very well balanced. Not bothering to read food labels is another of our bad habits. According to a recent American Dietetic Association survey, one in five African-Americans pays no attention to labels. How then are we supposed to know what nutrients we are—or aren't—getting?

For sisters who live in lower-income areas, bad shopping habits occur almost by default. What can we expect when access to large, well-stocked supermarkets is so limited in many black communities? Convenience stores, *bodegas,* and mom-and-pop shops are some sisters' only choices. Odds are you won't find a variety of produce, quality meats, or fresh fruit in these stores. They sell what sells best: processed food. The irony is that these high-in-calorie, low-in-nutrient corner-store foods typically cost more than fresh, better-quality items found in sprawling suburban supermarkets. Poor folks end up paying more and getting less. Trust us, cooking from scratch will save you money.

Why is fresh better? Because you can control the end result. Sure, pre-packaged is more convenient, but it may contain more salt, sugar, and fats than you need. Taking off pounds is so much harder when you're not in control of how your foods are prepared. Our advice? Make fresh foods your first choice, frozen your second. We know that's a difficult rule of thumb for you sisters who simply don't have a good supermarket nearby. Not to worry. We're going to give you an economical plan of action to stock a healthy, hearty, nutritious kitchen no matter where you live.

Smart Shopping Saves You Bucks

Stocking your refrigerator and cupboards with healthy foods, without breaking the bank, isn't as difficult as you might think. Sure, sisters who live close to a big supermarket will have more choices, but even those of you who need to buy groceries at the corner store have options.

Is there a farmers' market in your city? If so, make a special trip and buy in bulk. Farmers' markets, also known as green-markets in many areas, are wonderful, typically open-air venues filled with fresh fruits and vegetables that usually cost less than those in the store. Talk to your sister circle. Maybe they'll want to make a day at the greenmarket a regular outing—say, once a week. That way, you can all stock up on delicious, fresh produce while enjoying one another's company.

It may also be worth the gas for you and your sisterfriends to hit the supermarkets in neighboring communities two or three times a month. Yes, it may be out of the way, but it will give you the opportunity to supplement your weekly convenience-store groceries with the meats and produce you can't find near home. The bottom line is that sisters who live in poorer areas will have to make more of an effort to buy good foods. They aren't going to come to you; you have to go to them. But utilizing your sister circle will make it easier.

Gaining access to quality foods is half the battle. Once you're in the store, you have to make the right choices. Let's start with meats. Think lean. You want to choose meats that have a lower fat content. Instead of picking up that package of ground beef as you normally would, opt for extra-lean ground beef, ground round, or ground turkey. It may cost a bit more, but we're going to show you how to get more out of it. It's all about extending your dollar—buying the best foods you can, for the smallest amount you can, and then working those recipes until they yield the most meals possible.

Another smart way to save on meats: Befriend the store's butcher. By purchasing rump and loin roasts and having him cut them into chops and stew cubes, instead of buying them pre-packaged, you'll save money. Ask him to trim off the excess fat for you.

When buying chicken, stick to whole birds—they're cheaper and you'll get more out of them than if you buy, say, a package of chicken breasts. If you do opt for parts, buy the family packs and freeze whatever's left over for future meals.

Consider generic brands when buying staples like rice, pasta, beans, and cereal. You'll net big savings.

To save money on vegetables, skip the canned varieties and buy them fresh. Not only will they contain a greater amount of nutrients, they'll also cost less (you'll get more for your money). Frozen is your next-best bet for nutrition value. Worried that some frozen brand-names are out of your price range? Then stick to the store brands; they're usually cheaper and just as good. Remember, too, bagged isn't bad when it comes to potatoes. Bagged spuds tend to cost less than loose ones. The same principle holds true for oranges and apples.

Really want to trim your food bill? Then pay more attention to seasonings. As we've told you, black folks often opt for fatty meats because of the flavor. But jazzing up lean cuts, traditional greens, and other low-calorie healthful foods is easy if you have an arsenal of herbs and spices. Inexpensive staples like rice, pasta, and beans can be used as the bases of many meals, with a little meat added for taste (the less meat you use, the more dollars you save), and savory seasonings sprinkled in to bring forth all the wonderful flavor. Forget bland. The right spices can make any dish sing. So be sure to have more than salt, pepper, and garlic in your cabinets. Try tarragon, oregano, thyme, paprika, ginger, basil, cumin, curry, bay leaves, and any others that light your imagination.

Dining Out the Right Way

Even the most healthfully stocked kitchen won't make a difference if you chow down when you're not home, especially if you eat out often. And as a matter of fact, we do. According to "What We Eat in America," a 1995 USDA nationwide food-consumption survey, more than half—51 percent to be exact—of African-Americans eat away from home, most often in fast-food restaurants. McDonald's, Burger King, Taco Bell, Kentucky Fried Chicken—all of these places and a host of others offer fast, hot, relatively inexpensive meals that sisters can grab when they're on the go. Unfortunately, the foods we like best at these places tend to be higher in fat, salt, and cholesterol and lower in nutrients than the food we can eat at home. Let's be real. A burger, fries, and a soda can't begin to compare with a home-cooked meal of baked chicken, rice, and greens—or some other stick-to-your-ribs, good-for-you food. Maybe if you order the "healthier" fare that most fast-food places offer these days, say a grilled chicken sandwich (without mayo or cheese), a side salad, and a diet soda, it wouldn't be so bad. But how many of us really select that when Big Macs, Whoppers, and two-piece meals are calling our names? And let's not forget about super-sizing. Why buy regular when you can get gigantic? More for the money, right? Perhaps, if you don't mind shortchanging your health. Take a look at how a few typical fast-food items stack up:

Whopper	*French Fries (large)*
614 calories	682 calories
36 grams of total fat	19 grams of total fat
90 grams of cholesterol	42 grams of cholesterol

Add a soda and that comes out to a whole day's worth of calories in one meal! Fast-food joints aren't the only culprits, though. Nice, ambient, sit-down restaurants are full of keep-you-fat traps too. Who's going to pass up that basket of piping hot bread while waiting for dinner to arrive? We'll probably splurge too—on gooey desserts, fat-laden meals, and high-calorie cocktails. It's natural to want to treat yourself when you're out on the town. But keep this up and you're going to treat yourself to a few more pounds.

If you're going to the effort of filling your fridge and cupboards with good-for-you foods, why sabotage yourself by making poor choices away from home? There's nothing wrong with eating out. No one wants to brown-bag it every day, and Lord knows hardworking sisters owe themselves a night or two out enjoying nice restaurants. But if you expect to shed those pounds, you have to use the same sort of conscious decision making at a restaurant or fast-food joint that you use at home. So when eating out, keep these tips in mind:

- Think before you eat. Take time to consider whether you're making the best, most healthful choice.
- Ask how meats are prepared. Select entrées that are baked or broiled. If it's not prepared that way, make a special request. Skip fried foods.
- Have salad dressing and sauces served on the side, so that you can control how much is used.
- When presented with a basket of bread, it's okay to have a piece, just don't have it with so much butter. Reduce the amount you'd normally spread on; use one pat and make it last the whole meal.
- Make it easier on yourself—opt for foods with no sauce, gravy, or butter added.
- When having salad, nix the croutons, grated cheese, bacon bits, nuts, and other fattening add-ons. Stick to low-calorie dressing, or drizzle on balsamic vinegar and lemon juice.
- Itching for dessert? Choose something low-fat, such as fruit, ice milk, low-fat frozen yogurt, angel food cake, or fruit gelatin.
- Pass up super-size portions.
- Split big entrées with your husband or a friend.
- Switch from soda to water, unsweetened iced tea, or diet soda.
- At fast-food places, pick the healthier items on the menu— say, a grilled chicken sandwich. Ask for it plain, without the mayonnaise, dressing, or "secret sauce." Spread on some mustard instead.

The *Slim Down Sister* Food Plan

Rather than provide you with a rigid diet that stifles your food choices, we're simply going to tell you what types of foods to eat each day. After all, none of us wants to feel deprived or bullied. Losing weight and improving your health means changing your lifestyle. How can you do that if a restrictive diet forbids you to have cornbread or pork chops or mashed potatoes? As you'll see in the next chapter, you can have all that and more, as long as you prepare your meals the right way.

For now, however, let's focus on the food. While you will be able to enjoy the cuisine you love, we're not giving you the green light for a food free-for-all. You will have to adhere to some limits. The hard truth is, you have to cut back on what you eat (and work out too, of course) to lose weight. The more you weigh, the more you have to cut back. Don't worry, girlfriend. It's not as ominous as it sounds.

First of all, you should never eat less than 1,200 calories a day. That's downright dangerous, no matter what anyone else may tell you. Consume too few calories and your body *is* going to rebel. No question about it. "By any means necessary" doesn't apply to losing weight. You need enough fuel—sustenance—to keep your body active and your mind sharp. A physical and mental shutdown from eating too little isn't going to get you closer to your weight-loss goal. Remember, too, the point of all this isn't to look fly. It's to improve your health and cut your risk of obesity-related diseases. By following a severely restrictive diet, you're going to accomplish the very thing you're trying to avoid: poor health.

So when we say the more you weigh, the more you have to cut back, we're talking about realistic, doable, sustainable cutbacks—consuming 1,200 to 1,800 calories a day. That amount leaves you lots of room to maneuver. For some of you, getting to the 1,200-to-1,800-calorie range simply means trimming 500 or so calories from your daily intake (not really that hard to do). For other, heavier sisters, it may mean cutting as much as 2,000 or more calories from your daily intake.

How do we know this? It's easy to figure. Say you weigh 175 pounds right now. To maintain that weight you need to take in 2,625 calories a day. We're using the 15-calorie-per-pound rule of thumb. You multiply your weight by 15; the result is the number of calories you need each day for weight maintenance. For many sisters, cutting 500 to 750 calories a day, combined with moderate exercise, nets a 1- to 2-pound-per-week weight loss. But if you weigh, say, 250 pounds, you'll need to scale back more in order to slim down. Following the rule of thumb calculation, a 250-pound sister consumes 3,750 calories a day just to maintain her present weight. To get into our recommended 1,200-to-1,800-calorie range, she'd have to trim at least 1,950 calories from her daily diet.

Having a choice in how you go about trimming those calories makes things easier and allows you to stick to your new eating plan without feeling deprived. We've broken down the plan into three sections: 1,200 calories a day, 1,500 calories a day, and 1,800 calories a day. Select the one that feels right for you, or try different combinations. As long as you don't go over the 1,800 limit you'll be fine.

Each plan tells you how many servings or ounces to have of each type of food (as outlined on the Soul Food Pyramid), and how many carbohydrates, proteins, and fats to have each day. Make copies of the recall sheet on page 105 and use them to keep track. First, fill in the last row of the chart on each sheet—the recommended totals for your chosen plan (2 milks per day, 3 fruits per day, 6 breads per day, and so on—whatever your chosen plan calls for). Then, whenever you eat something, jot down the time of day, what you ate, how much you had, and how it was prepared. Next, check off the appropriate category in the columns on the right-hand side of the chart—M=Milk, V=Vegetable, FR=Fruit, B=Bread, MT=Meat, and F=Fat. Not sure what constitutes a serving? Check the Soul Food Pyramid for quick reference.

You'll notice that the fats category on the Soul Food Pyramid simply encourages you to eat fats "sparingly." However, we know that you may need more specific advice. So, when eating fats, keep these guidelines in mind.

One serving of fat equals:

1 teaspoon stick or tub margarine/butter
1 tablespoon diet margarine
1 teaspoon mayonnaise
1 tablespoon reduced-fat/lite mayonnaise
1 tablespoon salad dressing
2 tablespoons low-cal salad dressing

1 slice bacon

1 tablespoon cream cheese

2 tablespoons fat-free cream cheese

1 teaspoon corn, safflower, soybean, canola, olive, or peanut oil

½ ounce chitterlings

You'll see that we've made room for snacks, too. They're built right into each plan. Say you've decided to follow the 1,200-calorie plan. You don't have to have both servings of bread and that serving of fruit in the morning if you don't want to. You can use them as a midmorning or afternoon snack instead. That's how we want you to approach each plan when it comes to noshing. Save servings of different foods here and there and use them as snacks any time of day. Thought you'd have to give that up, didn't you? Well, you don't. Snacks can be part of a healthy weight-loss plan *if* you eat the right things (low in calories, high in nutrients), and remember that moderation is key.

Why do we snack? For several reasons: because we're always on the go due to crazy work schedules and often don't have time for three squares a day; out of habit or routine; because we're bored, anxious, lonely, upset, or feeling some other extreme emotion; some of us even munch simply because we're happy. Whatever the reason, snacking can put a serious dent in your efforts to get fit, especially if you nosh on empty-calorie snacks (remember, low-fat doesn't necessarily mean low in calories), and eat out-of-control portions. Keep those snacks in check, though, and you can easily make them part of your healthy eating plan.

A nutritious, filling snack takes the edge off your appetite between meals, which means you won't overdo when you sit down for lunch and dinner. Good snacks can also help curb nighttime refrigerator raids—a big problem for lots of us. You know the drill: You do great all day long, but as soon as the sun sets and you're snuggled up in front of the television, you get a craving for something sweet, or salty, or whatever your particular soft spot happens to be for. With our plan, you won't have to sit there fighting with yourself about whether or not to indulge. Just refer to your chosen plan, see how many snacks you have left, then select something that fits within the guidelines. Here are a few tips and suggestions to help you choose your snacks wisely:

- It's not surprising that many of us crave goodies from the top of the food pyramid—cookies, chips, soda, candy, ice cream, and the like. When you feel the urge to snack, however, it's far healthier to select foods from other parts of the pyramid.
- Always practice portion control so that your snacks don't get out of hand. Use a small plate or bowl. Share it with someone else. Divvy up snack foods into single-serving portions. And avoid any on-the-run foods labeled "Biggie," "Jumbo," "Supersize," or "Big Gulp."
- Make sure snacks contain fewer than 100 calories apiece.
- If you're the type of sister who eats lunch late, or who lets more than four hours go between breakfast and your next hearty meal, have a midmorning snack and make it a good one—opt for a small whole-grain bagel, a slice of toast, or a small muffin, with a low-fat milk product and some fresh fruit.
- For afternoon and evening snacks, pretzels, celery sticks and carrots, fruit, or half of a tuna sandwich made with low-fat/low-cal mayo are all better choices than a quickie candy bar.
- Drink low-calorie or no-calorie fluids with your snacks. Try water. You should be drinking lots of it every day anyway. Why not get more H_2O daily by having a big glass or two with every snack?
- More healthy snack picks: baked tortilla chops with salsa, fat-free frozen yogurt, graham crackers, fruit bars. Fruits such as bananas, grapes, apples, and orange slices (toss them in a plastic Baggie) are good commuter snacks—great taste, less mess.

Our plan gives you permission to eat well and feel satisfied. If you need a jump-start with your menus, check out the samples that follow the food plans. Want more? You'll find slimmed-down soul-food recipes in Appendix B.

Daily Food Plan

	1,200 cal.	1,500 cal.	1,800 cal.
Carbohydrates (grams)	154	194	224
Protein (grams)	60	75	93
Fat (grams)	37	48	59
Morning			
Milk servings	1	1	1
Fruit servings	1	1	1
Bread servings	2	2	3
Meat, total ounces	1	1	2
Fat servings	1	2	2
Noon			
Milk servings	0	1	1
Vegetable servings	1	1	2
Fruit servings	1	1	1
Bread servings	2	2	2
Meat, total ounces	1	2	2
Fat servings	1	1	2
Evening			
Milk servings	1	0	0
Vegetable servings	1	2	2
Fruit servings	1	1	1
Bread servings	1	2	3
Meat, total ounces	2	2	2
Fat servings	1	1	2

SAMPLE MENUS

1,200 Calories	1,200 Calories	1,500 Calories
Breakfast	**Breakfast**	**Breakfast**
½ cup orange juice 1 small bagel (about 2 ozs.) 2 tsp. fat-free cream cheese coffee 1 cup skim milk	½ cup orange-pinapple juice 1 cup dry cereal 1 cup skim milk 1 slice whole wheat toast coffee	1 banana 1 scrambled egg ½ cup grits 1 slice whole wheat toast w/1 tsp. margarine 1 cup skim milk coffee
Lunch	**Lunch**	**Lunch**

turkey sandwich
  1 oz. smoked turkey
  1 oz. low-fat cheese
  2 slices whole wheat
  bread
  1 tsp. mayo
1 medium apple
low-cal drink
	chef's salad w/1 oz. of
	  turkey and ham, 1 oz. of
	  low-fat cheese
	2 tsp. low-cal dressing
	small whole wheat roll
	1 medium pear
	low-cal drink
		6-inch sub or hero roll
		  w/2 oz meat (turkey, ham)
		1 tbsp. reduced-fat mayo
		1 orange
		low-cal drink

Dinner	**Dinner**	**Dinner**

3 oz. baked chicken
½ cup yellow rice
½ cup green beans
tossed salad w/2 tsp
  low-cal dressing
low-cal drink
 	
Snack:
  1 cup watermelon
	3 oz. grilled pork chop
	½ cup garlic mashed
	  potatoes
	1 cup vegetable medley
	Caesar salad w/2 tsp.
	  low-cal dressing
	small whole wheat roll
	low-cal drink
	
	Snack:
	  1 cup fresh fruit salad
		½ cup spaghetti
		  noodles w/½ cup
		  meat sauce
		1 cup broccoli
		tossed salad w/low-cal
		  dressing
		roll w/1 tsp. margarine
		low-cal drink
		
		Snack:
		  ½ cup low-fat frozen
		  yogurt w/1cup
		  strawberries

1,500 Calories	1,800 Calories	1,800 Calories
Breakfast	**Breakfast**	**Breakfast**

½ cup orange sections
2 waffles
1 slice bacon
2 tbsp. low-cal syrup
1 cup skim milk
coffee
	½ cup orange sections
	1 cup grits
	1 egg
	1 slice whole wheat bread
	2 tsp. margarine
	1 cup skim milk
		½ cup orange juice
		2 slices whole wheat
		  bread
		1 oz. low-fat cheese
		  (sliced)
		1 tbsp. diet margarine
		1 cup skim milk
		coffee

Lunch	**Lunch**	**Lunch**

1 cup chicken noodle soup
½ cup egg salad
2 slices whole wheat bread
1 cup cantaloupe
1 cup skim milk
	2 slices whole wheat bread
	2 oz. turkey breast
	1 oz. low-fat cheese
	lettuce and tomatoes
	1 tbsp. reduced-calorie
	  mayo
	1 apple
	low-cal drink
		large tossed salad
		  w/tomatoes, carrots,
		  and raw vegetables
		1 oz. ham
		1 boiled egg
		1 cup beef noodle soup
		1 small whole wheat roll
		2 tbsp. diet salad dressing
		1 cup melon

Dinner	**Dinner**	**Dinner**

3 oz. grilled chicken
1 small baked sweet potato
1 cup steamed cabbage
1 piece cornbread
low-cal drink
 	
Snack:
  1 cup strawberries
  w/lite whipped topping
	3 oz. baked chicken
	1 cup brown rice
	1 cup cooked broccoli
	tossed salad w/1 tbsp. diet
	  dressing
	small whole wheat roll
	  w/1 tsp. margarine
	low-cal drink
	
	Snack:
	  diet Jell-O w/½ cup
	  fruit packed in own juice
		3 oz. grilled pork chop
		  w/½ cup pineapple chunks
		  in teriyaki sauce
		1 medium baked
		  sweet potato
		1 cup green beans
		1 small dinner roll
		2 tbsp. diet margarine
		low-cal drink
		
		Snack:
		  ½ cup baked custard

SAMPLE RECALL SHEET

Time	Food/Beverage	Amount/How Prepared	M	V	FR	B	MT	F
7 AM	egg	1 scrambled					√	
	Whole wheat toast	1 slice w/pat butter				√		√
	Orange juice	½ cup			√			
1 PM	Turkey w/lettuce and mustard	2 oz.		√			√	
	Whole wheat bread	2 slices				√√		
	Salad	small w/low-cal dressing		√				√
	Apple	small		√				
	Skim milk	1 cup	√					
6 PM	Baked chicken	3 oz./baked					√	
	Collards	1 cup/boiled w/smoked turkey		√				
	Sweet potato	1 baked		√				
	Dinner roll	1 small				√		
	Diet soda	1 can (12 oz.)						
	Fruit salad	1 cup		√				
8 PM	Graham crackers	2				√		
	Skim milk	1 cup	√					
Your Totals			2	4	3	5	3	2
Recommended Totals for the Chosen Plan			2	3	3	8	5	4

Notes:

RECALL SHEET

Time	Food/Beverage	Amount/How Prepared	M	V	FR	B	MT	F
Your Totals								
Recommended Totals for the Chosen Plan								

Notes:

Sister to Sister

Tonya Chavis, a thirty-six-year-old massage therapist from
   Freehold, New Jersey
Current weight: 120 pounds
Amount lost: 32 pounds

I've lost weight twice. The first time was eight years ago
when my husband and I first moved to Freehold. I wasn't
working then, and I didn't know anyone in our new town,
so I sat at home, watched my soaps, and nibbled. Before I
knew it I was about 30 pounds overweight. It kind of
sneaked up on me.

I started exercising and changed my eating habits, but I
was addicted to the scale. I'd get on it constantly. I was
playing head games with the scale and driving myself
crazy, so I finally got rid of it. I just went by how my clothes
fit and how I felt. And you know what? That's when I
started losing weight.

Two years later I got pregnant. After I had my son I
wanted to work out right away, but because I'd had a C-
section my doctor told me I had to wait two months. By
the time I could exercise, I had 32 pounds to lose. This
time around, though, I also had a child, which places a lot
of demands on your time.

I started walking in the park with the baby. I'd push him
in his stroller. I joined a gym, too, and took a few aerobics
classes, but that just wasn't working for me. I had to get a
babysitter, drive to the gym, then go back and pick up my
child, and so on. It was a hassle and very time-consuming.
It was so much easier to do things that included the baby,
like walking in the park.

I didn't go on a "diet," either. I was simply more aware
of what went in my mouth. I put more thought into it. I ate
fruit as a snack and as dessert. I increased the vegetables

in my meals and stuck to chicken and fish for the most part. I also made subtle changes, like having my coffee black instead of putting cream in it, and not putting sugar in my iced tea anymore. These small changes were fairly easy to make because I didn't have to do everything all at once. When you start to cut out sugar you find that you don't really need or crave it. I didn't tell myself that I was never going to eat cake or ice cream again. If I felt like having it, I'd pay attention and have a small amount. Even now, when my family goes out to dinner, we'll have dessert, but we'll ask for one dessert with three spoons.

I found that by eating more fruit and vegetables, I ate less junk because I was already satisfied. Fruit and veggies keep you full longer than a bag of potato chips ever will. By chewing on something like a carrot you satisfy that chewing urge. You can't just pop a carrot in your mouth, two chews and it's gone.

I like to have soul food, but I know that I need to limit myself and make sure it's prepared as healthfully as it can be. You can have your greens and your sweet potatoes. It's all in how you fix them.

My main thing is to always have a salad. Even if I stop by McDonald's, I'll get the salad instead of the other stuff.

It sounds so cliché, but it really is true. You have to take it one day at a time. When I wake up in the morning, I say to myself, "I'm going to make healthy choices today." If I blow it at breakfast, I still have the rest of the day to put good things in my body. I always try to remember that. I also remind myself of where I've been and what I've accomplished. All I have to ask myself is, "Do you want to lose 32 pounds all over again or do you want to maintain your weight right now?" I think you know the answer. That one question helps me stay on track.

CHAPTER 6

✣

Out of the Frying Pan

There are three little words that every sister who loves good soul food knows to be true: Fat equals flavor. We don't go around consciously trying to figure out ways to add fat to our meals. It just happens. That's the way we cook. That's the way we eat. Fat is built right into the foods we consume every day: meat, chicken, cheese, eggs, milk, and so on. It's the good stuff that makes our cooking sing: the butter that melts in our grits, the shortening that pops so deliciously as we fry up some chicken or fish, the ham hocks that season our greens just right. And it's the invisible addition to the snack foods we munch: chips, dough-nuts, fries, and the like. As good as it tastes, however, the truth is that too much dietary fat can be dangerous. Not only can it lead to obesity, a high-fat diet can also put you at increased risk for cardiovascular disease, diabetes, and cancer.

But before you throw out all of your butter and cooking oil, listen up. We're not saying your have to banish fat from your life. In fact, having some fat in your diet is essential. But in order to improve your health and drop those pounds, you do need to make sure you're consuming the right type of fat in the right amounts. Make a real effort to do that, and soon those three little words will become four: *Less* fat equals flavor.

The Facts About Fat

High-fat, low-fat, saturated fat, fatty acids. With all of these fat terms floating around, is it any wonder many sisters can't make head nor tail of the whole business? Just what the heck *is* fat anyway? To put it simply, fats are nutrients that help provide the body with energy. (Every gram of fat supplies nine calories.) They are made up of carbon, hydrogen, and a little oxygen. When you put all three elements together, you get what's called fatty acids. If the fatty acids contain all the hydrogen possible, they are *saturated*. If some of the hydrogen is missing, then the fatty acids are *unsaturated*. Here's where things get a little complicated. You've heard of polyunsaturated and monounsaturated, right? Well, when fatty acids are missing only one hydrogen atom on that carbon-hydrogen-oxygen chain we told you about, they're *monounsaturated*. If they're missing two or more hydrogen atoms, they're *polyunsaturated*.

Right about now you're probably scratching your head, thinking "Huh?" Let's break it down. What's the real difference between saturated and unsaturated fat—aside from how much hydrogen they contain? In a word, cholesterol. As you've no doubt heard, having high cholesterol puts you at greater risk for heart disease. Here's how it works: There's a fat molecule in your body called a lipoprotein that carries cholesterol around in the blood. High levels of low-density lipoproteins (LDLs) are considered "bad" because they head straight to your arteries and block them up, which can lead to heart disease. High-density lipoproteins (HDLs), on the other hand, are seen as "good" because they carry cholesterol to the liver for excretion, thus protecting you against heart disease.

As you can see, fats have a funny way of being both good for you and bad for you. That's why it's so important to be up on your fat facts.

The Good, the Bad, and the Downright Ugly

Here's some news you're sure to like: A certain amount of dietary fat is actually good for you. Not only does it energize your body (fat stores provide a constant source of extra energy when you need it most), it also helps your body absorb fat-soluble vitamins A, D, E, and K. Fat cushions your organs and protects them from injury, serves as an insulator to help you stay warm on cold days, and satisfies hunger by making you feel full after eating. Most sisters want too much of a good thing, though, and that's when they start to get into trouble. You only need a little bit of fat to stay healthy—no more then 30 percent of your daily total caloric intake. But given black folks' typical diet, many of us end up eating far more than that. You have to cut back on the fat if you want to lose weight. Just keep in mind that while all fats are high in calories, some are better than others healthwise. Here's how to tell friend from foe.

Saturated fats (reduce them). Found mostly in animal products (including dairy foods such as cheese and eggs), lard, and tropical oils (coconut, palm, and palm kernel). An easy way to recognize unsaturated fats: They are firm or solid at room temperature. The harder the fat, the more saturated it is: for example, butter, cheese, and the fat in meats are all highly saturated.

Monounsaturated fats (a healthier alternative). Found in canola, peanut, and olive oils, and in avocados and some nuts. These fats are liquid at room temperature.

Polyunsaturated fats (another good bet). These fats are found in vegetable oils such as safflower, soybean, and sunflower oils. Seafood is high in polyunsaturated fat, too. Like their monounsaturated cousins, polyunsaturated fats are also liquid at room temperature.

Trans-fatty acids (cut back). Found in margarine, solid vegetable shortening, and various snack foods. These fatty acids are made during the process of hydrogenation, in which hydrogen is added to liquid fats in order to turn them into solids. (Think of a tub of margarine, for example—it didn't start out that way.) Hydrogenation extends a product's shelf-life, but also makes fats more saturated. A product that contains *trans*-fatty acids will have partially hydrogenated oil listed in its ingredients.

Omega-3 fatty acids (the good-for-your-heart fat). Found in seafood; tuna, mackerel, and salmon are particularly good sources of Omega-3. These fatty acids, which are high in poly-unsaturated fat, protect your heart and help prevent blood clots.

Why Fry Is a Four-Letter Word

Remember your mama's fried chicken? The way she used to drop each piece into a brown paper bag of seasoned flour, shake it up, then gently place each one in a cast-iron skillet hissing with the sound of bubbling hot grease? She'd tell you to "get from that stove" so you wouldn't catch a pop of grease. You just couldn't wait. Nothing tasted better than mama's fried chicken, whether hot off the paper towel or plucked cold from the refrigerator the next day.

Traditions die hard, and chances are your own children wait with wide-eyed anticipation as you fry your chicken today, just the way your mother did—with that brown paper bag, big black skillet, and warnings to stand back from the stove. What in the world could be wrong with fixing meals the same way our parents and grandparents did? Well, that all depends. How much of their food was fried? If your family is like generations of other black families in this country, the answer is probably too much.

We like fried food, plain and simple. Now, if we ate it only once in a while, there wouldn't be a problem. But black folks eat more fried foods than we should. The fault with frying? Fat, fat,

and more fat. Deep frying and pan frying—two black-folk faves—
are definitely not the ways to go if you're trying to eat healthfully.
Sure, it tastes good, but every time you fry, you either add fat or
allow the food to cook in its own fat. Remember, each gram of fat
contains nine calories. So by frying your food, you're unwittingly
loading up on calories. Before you know it, those 1,200, 1,500, or
1,800 calories that are supposed to see you through breakfast,
lunch, dinner, and snacks have been nearly eaten up in one or
two meals.

Don't believe us? Then consider this: One 3-ounce piece of
fried chicken has 14.7 grams of fat and 226 calories. That's one
piece! If you take that same piece of chicken and "fry" it in the
oven, you save more than half the fat and nearly as much in calories. One 3-ounce piece of oven-fried chicken has a mere 5.5
grams of fat and only 117 calories. That's a mighty big difference.
Not only do you put the brakes on health risks by preparing your
meals in a more low-fat fashion, you'll also give yourself more
room for other tasty foods. Why spend the bulk of your calories
on fat when you can spend it on other foods that will fill you up
and leave you satisfied?

Let's take a look at a typical dinner, one many black folks are
likely to eat on a regular basis. Compare the usual preparation
method and the low-fat alternative.

Typical African-American Meal

	Fat	Calories
1 piece of fried chicken (3 oz.)	14.7	226
½ cup macaroni and cheese	14.2	353
½ cup pork-seasoned collard greens	28	280
Sliced tomatoes w/mayonnaise	5	67
1 piece of cornbread with butter	17	182
1 piece of sweet-potato pie	9.7	283
	88.6 gm.	1,391

Low-Fat Alternative

	Fat	Calories
1 piece of oven-fried chicken (3 oz.)	5.5	117
½ cup macaroni and cheese made with low-fat cheese and an egg substitute such as Eggbeaters	6.2	234
½ cup collard greens seasoned with smoked turkey parts	5.3	159
Sliced tomatoes with low-fat mayonnaise	2.1	43
1 piece of cornbread made with skim milk and Eggbeaters	7.0	150
1 slice of low-fat sweet-potato pie	5.5	170
	31.6 gm.	873

Clearly, the low-fat alternative saves you fat and calories. Best of all, it tastes just as good as its high-fat cousin. With a few minor adjustments, all of your meals can be healthful and satisfying.

We know we may be asking a lot of you. Change is never easy. But girlfriend, if you'll simply give our way a chance, you'll see that low-fat cooking can be as delicious as the high-fat method. The secret is in the preparation. We're not going to have you toss a piece of chicken in the oven, turn up the heat, then eat whatever comes out. Girl, please. We wouldn't want to eat that bland, old, tired piece of chicken either. The recipes and tips we'll be sharing with you make use of a cornucopia of herbs, spices and seasonings that will bring out all the down-home flavor you love. (Check out the Slimmed-Down Soul-Food Recipes in Appendix B.) For now, though, let's focus on the method.

A Better Way

You know that shortening you like so much? Shove it in the back of the fridge. (Hey, out of sight, out of mind.) The bacon grease you swear by? Toss it right on out. (You knew *something* had to go.) Welcome to a better way of cooking. Full of flava? Yes indeed. Full of fat? No way.

First order of business: Rethink the way you prepare your meats. There are a host of cooking methods that will leave meat, fish, and poultry moist, succulent, and tasty. So don't be so quick to reach for the frying pan. Instead, try the following fat-saving methods.

Bake. Great for poultry, meat, and fish. Simply add a bit of water or fat-free, low-sodium flavored broth to the pan, cover with aluminum foil, and pop it in the oven. For extra flavor, toss a few onion slices or other seasonings into the pan before baking.

Braise. Pan-brown meat or poultry using a little nonstick cooking spray, then add a small amount of liquid. Cover the pot and slowly bake in the oven or simmer on top of the stove. Your meat will come out juicy and flavorful. An additional fat-blaster: Braise the meat ahead of time, then refrigerate. The fat will congeal, making it easy to skim off before reheating. Try braising vegetables, too.

Broil. Another tasty low-fat way to make fish, meat, and poultry. Broil your meats on a rack in a broiler pan; the fat drips right off. Broiled meats can burn easily, so keep an eye on them as they cook.

Grill. Similar to broiling, but the coals add a nice smoky flavor. You can grill just about anything—meats, fish, poultry, even veggies. (Try a vegetable-and-diced-meat combo kebab.) Spice things up by marinating meats before grilling.

Poach. Simmer a pan of liquid (water will do fine) on top of the stove. Place your chicken or fish in the pan (make sure the food is immersed in the water) and cover. You can add a dash of herbs and spices to the liquid to boost the flavor. As your fish or poultry cooks, make sure the water simmers gently, but doesn't boil—this helps ensure tenderness. After removing the cooked food from the pan, add puréed vegetables to the remaining liquid to make a light sauce—a nice complement to poached fish or poultry.

Roast. Set meat or poultry on a rack in the roasting pan so the fat can drain off. A fat-fighting tip: Don't baste your meat with pan juices; opt for a fat-free liquid instead. Try a richly flavored broth—make sure it's defatted and low in sodium.

Sauté. This technique traditionally calls for frying food in some amount of fat or oil. Grab a nonstick pan and you'll only need a few drops of oil to sauté poultry, fish, or vegetables. Better yet, use a nonstick vegetable spray or a little bit of broth.

Steam. A quick and easy way to prepare vegetables and fish. Just place food in a colander or steamer basket over boiling water and cover. In about ten minutes or less, it's done. In addition to its no-added-fat benefit, steaming also allows food to retain much of its vitamins, minerals, color, and flavor.

Stir-fry. The high temperature and constant stirring keep stir-fried foods from sticking to the pan, so you won't need very much oil at all. Use a very hot wok or skillet to stir-fry small cut pieces of poultry, meat, seafood, and vegetables. You'll find that your food cooks quite quickly with this method.

Wean yourself from frying by giving these new cooking methods a go several times a week. Where else can your cooking techniques use an overhaul? Are you making the best choices in meats? How about with ingredients? When a recipe calls for an egg, do you just crack one open or do you stop to consider a healthier alternative? Always take a moment to ask yourself, "What's the healthiest choice?" Think before you cook—make this your new motto in the kitchen.

Quick Tips to Remember

- Rather than frying your chicken or pork chops, try baking and grilling them instead to cut down on fat.
- Instead of adding ham hocks to greens such as collards, or to dry beans try smoked skinless turkey or chicken broth. You'll be pumping up the flavor, not the fat.
- Have a taste for potato salad? Go ahead and make some. But

instead of using regular mayonnaise and a couple of hard-boiled eggs, opt for low-fat mayo and use fewer eggs.

- No need to give up cornbread. Simply make it with only the egg white or an egg substitute, and use canola oil. The result? You got it—less fat.
- At breakfast, replace those old standbys—bacon, sausage, and ham—with equally tasty (but less fatty) turkey products, Canadian bacon, and lean ham.
- One of sisters' all-time favorites, macaroni and cheese, is loaded with fat. You can make it more healthful by using low-fat cheese and low-fat milk.

Make Use of the Microwave

If you only use your microwave when you need to warm up something, then it's time to look at it in a new way. The microwave is much more than a re-heating machine. It can be a very useful tool for pressed-for-time sisters like you who want to eat right without a lot of hassle. Microwave cooking is fast, easy, and—best of all—requires no added fat. Just make sure to go with foods that cook well in moist heat: vegetables, fish, chicken, ground meat, and soups. Another boon to your health: because you use less water when cooking in the microwave, foods retain more of their vitamins.

When the Old Way Is the Best Way

Believe it or not, when it comes to healthy cooking, tradition sometimes wins out. Even though you may have to trade in your frying pan for a roasting pan now and then to lose weight, there are two tried-and-true soul-food techniques that actually serve you well: one-pot stewing and barbecuing.

Culturally speaking, stewing and barbecuing are both vital

parts of African-American cuisine. One-pot meals date back to the days of slavery, when our ancestors would often place a pot of vegetables and other ingredients out in the field, where it would stew all day as they toiled. When the sun set, the dinner meal was done. Similarly, the traditional summer barbecues we enjoy so much evolved from cooking techniques of the past. The African method of roasting meats in pits dug into the ground gave rise to the backyard grilling of today.

How can you eat savory stew and BBQ and still lose weight? First of all, since one-pot stews include lots of vegetables, you'll be chowing down on foods that are actually good for you. You can boost the healthfulness by making sure your stew is chock-full of assorted veggies. Although one-pot meals require a lengthy amount of cooking time, which can strip vegetables of many of their vitamins, they all end up in the stew liquid. Ladle up the juices when you fill your bowl and you'll still get the benefit of those vital nutrients.

BBQ takes a little more effort. Barbecue grilling is a healthy way to cook food because it allows the fat to drip off the meat and onto the coals. (Better there than in you.) The problem arises when sisters select high-fat meats to place on the grill. Barbecue spareribs sound familiar to you? By trimming as much fat as possible from the meat before grilling, you'll help reduce the amount of fat you consume. You should also select the leanest cuts of meat and try out less-fatty alternatives. Don't be afraid to experiment with something new. For example, beef short ribs contain less fat than traditional spareribs. Throw a few of those on the grill for a change. Brush on some tangy sauce and they'll taste just as mouth-watering as the ones you're used to. Don't forget about barbecued chicken either; it's another good choice for the grill—just remember to remove the skin before cooking or eating.

Kicking the Salt Habit

When you're preparing food, do you use salt as a major ingredient, liberally sprinkling it in with other seasonings as you cook? When you sit down at the table, do you automatically reach for the salt shaker, before you've even tasted the food? When snack attacks hit, do you crave chips, crackers, or some other salty treat? If this sounds like you, join the club. Many of us are "addicted" to salt. It's become something of a staple for black folks. Not sure if you're in a salt trap? Then try a little experiment: Consciously keep track of your sodium intake for one day. Every time you reach for the salt shaker, jot it down. If you add lots of salt as you cook, take note. Check product labels for the amount of sodium in all of the foods you eat that day, and write that down too. By the end of the day you may be quite surprised.

Indeed, 25 percent of the sodium we consume comes from the salt shaker or from the sodium-rich ingredients we add to food. That's not to mention the fact that almost all foods contain sodium naturally or get some added during processing. Some of the biggest salt culprits are processed foods, cheese, breads and cereals, cured meats, snack foods, pickles, canned soup, and frozen dinners. Most of us take in a whopping 5,000 to 7,000 milligrams of sodium a day, when we should be keeping it closer to the 3,000-to-4,000-milligram mark—that is, if we're free of hypertension and cardiac disease. Those of us who do have either of these conditions should keep our sodium intake under 2,000 milligrams a day.

Why do we love salt so much? Many black folks would say it's because food tastes too bland without it—or so we think. The truth is, salt is an acquired taste, one that likely develops in childhood. By the time we become adults, we're so accustomed to the flavor of salt that foods just don't taste right without it.

We're not doing ourselves any favors, though, because salt plays an important role in hypertension, a disease that now affects sisters in record numbers. Nearly one-third of black women have high blood pressure, according to the National Center for Health Statistics. And one in five of us dies from it every year, estimates the American Medical Association.

To truly understand how salt is connected to high blood pressure, you have to take a look at it as a compound. Sodium is a mineral that helps regulate the body's water balance, maintain normal heart rhythm, conduct nerve impulses, and contract muscles. Obviously, we need some sodium to keep our bodies running smoothly, but we don't need all that much. Any excess is taken care of by our kidneys, which get rid of it in our urine. In a sister who's salt-sensitive, however, that excess sodium isn't eliminated. Her kidneys hold on to it, causing her body to retain water. When that happens, her blood pressure goes up. And as we've told you before, hypertension can lead to congestive heart failure, stroke, or kidney damage.

If you're a salt lover, reducing the amount you eat can be a real boon to your health, whether you have high blood pressure or not. If you are already hypertensive, cutting back on salt can help bring the disease under control. If you're one of the fortunate sisters who doesn't suffer from high blood pressure, ridding yourself of salt overuse may help keep you from getting it. Either way, an African-American woman who's overweight would do well to reduce her salt intake, since obesity in and of itself is a contributing factor to high blood pressure. By scaling back the sodium, you take one of those risk factors out of the mix. You give yourself a health edge—and sisters need as much of that as they can get.

Kicking the salt habit is all about substitution. You don't just wake up one morning and say, "I'm going to stop eating salt." Cold turkey is not the way to go. And why should you? You can still get the flavor and zest of salt from other sodium-free products.

Getting over a salt craving is like anything else involved with losing weight and improving your health—you can't deprive yourself. That approach doesn't work because you get angry and fed-up, and pretty soon you give in. Even if you can develop the mettle to stick it out, psychologically you'll be categorizing certain foods as "bad," period. The message you'll be sending yourself is *I can't have it or anything like it.* Who wants to hear that? When you're changing your lifestyle—which is exactly what you're trying to do—adopting that kind of mindset hinders your progress because you're not allowing yourself any choices. The more choice you have, the more successful you'll be in the long run. Why do you think so many sisters who've lost weight put it all back on (and often more) later? Because they gave up too many of the foods they loved. They used a hard-core approach, depriving themselves of favorite foods and never taking the time to find good substitutes or alternatives.

So all of you salt lovers, take heart. There is a way for you to fulfill that craving without putting your health in harm's way. You can't do anything about the sodium that's in foods naturally, except to eat less of those particular foods—and that's certainly one of the things you should do. But you can take an even more active approach with the sodium you add to food yourself. Experiment with different herbs and spices to give foods the zip they'd normally get from salt. (Odds are, your dishes will come away with even more bite and tang.)

There are plenty of tasty salt-free spices that can add an extra dimension to your cooking: Chinese 5 spice, Mrs. Dash, jerk rubs, curry blends, Spike seasonings, and many more. You can also add dry herbs and spices to liquid ingredients when cooking.

These days, you'll find all sorts of fresh and dried herbs at the supermarket. When buying fresh herbs, make sure leaves are moist and fresh, with no signs of wilting or decay. Store them in the refrigerator and they should keep for about a week. It's best to add fresh herbs toward the end of cooking time.

Dried herbs and spices can begin to lose flavor several months after the jar has been opened. Test for freshness by crushing a bit in your hand then taking a whiff. If it doesn't have its distinctive scent, then it's time to throw it out. You can keep dried herbs and spices fresh longer by storing them in the fridge. An easy rule of thumb to keep in mind when substituting dried herbs for fresh: One teaspoon of dried for every tablespoon of fresh.

Not sure which herbs and spices go best with which foods? This quick listing will get you started.

When cooking	Try using
Beef	basil, rosmary, bay leaf, thyme
Chicken	ginger, sage, tarragon
Fish	basil, dill, fennel, ginger, oregano, paprika
Pork	cayenne pepper, clove, rosemary
Shrimp	basil, dill, ginger
Collards	garlic, hot pepper flakes
Green beans	basil, clove, dill, sage
Lima beans	sage, savory
Peas	basil, mint, oregano, tarragon, thyme
Spinach	marjoram, nutmeg, rosemary
Squash and sweet potatoes	allspice, cinnamon, clove, ginger, thyme
Tomatoes	basil, bay leaf, clove, nutmeg, oregano
Pasta	basil, chives, marjoram, oregano, saffron
Rice	cumin, fennel, saffron
White potatoes	basil, caraway, chives, dill, parsley
Legumes	basil, coriander, oregano, rosemary, savory, thyme

Tips to Remember

- Take the salt shaker off the table. If you have to keep getting up to use it, you'll be less likely to bother.
- Taste foods first before automatically adding salt. We're so conditioned to salting our meals that we don't take the time to find out if they really need it.
- Cut back on salt gradually. Don't try to make a major change all at once. Taking it slow will make things easier.
- When you get the urge to have a salty snack such as chips or nuts, grab a piece of fresh fruit or some vegetables instead. Always stock your kitchen with assorted fruit, and keep baggies of raw veggies such as carrots and celery washed, chopped, and ready to munch.
- Make it a habit to read the sodium content on food labels. Be a more selective shopper.
- Try liquid smoke. This product (available at supermarkets) adds a nice smoky taste to dry beans. You can also mix liquid smoke with a little olive oil and brush it over your chicken or pork for extra oomph.
- Another salt saver: As soon as you purchase meats from the grocery store, marinate them with salt-free spices in a Ziploc bag, then place the meats in the freezer. When you're ready to cook them they'll be full of flavor.

Sister to Sister
✕◇✕◇✕◇✕◇✕

Cheryl Wilson, a forty-year-old accounts-receivable supervisor who lives in New York, New York
Current weight: 200 pounds
Amount lost: 55 pounds

I've always been prone to picking up weight. I'd gain some, then lose some. Gain some, then lose some. I tried

Herbalife and Dick Gregory, but when it was over I'd go right back to my regular way of eating and re-gain the weight. I'd yo-yo. I'm not a junk food eater. I just like to eat food. And I used to eat in abundance, especially white-flour products—bread, pasta, macaroni and cheese. I over-ate. Two or three helpings was nothing unusual for me.

I was in trouble. I knew that if I kept eating that way that I was going to be in danger, physically and emotion-ally, for the rest of my life. So I prayed. I went to the One who created me and asked Him for advice. After that I was able to make the decision to change my life. What-ever it took for me not to be in this place, I would do. The trade-off of feeling good and having a healthy body in-stead of overeating and feeling miserable was an easy one to make.

I'll admit, I did want to look good, but I was more con-cerned with my health. If I'd only wanted to look good, I probably would have gone on another one of those fad di-ets. But I knew I needed to make permanent changes. The things in my life that I could control, I wanted to control.

I bought a juicer and started drinking lots of fresh juices. I noticed immediately that it helped to curb my cravings. I also cut out white-flour products and switched to wheat-flour products and grains—wheat bread, wheat pasta. I began eating more organic foods, too. Once I'd changed the types of foods I was eating, the pounds started coming off slowly. I wasn't consuming as many high-calorie foods, but I was still eating a great deal. Por-tion size continued to be a problem for me. Even if you change what you eat, many of your old habits don't stop. You have to deal with those separately. Just because you're consuming healthy foods, it doesn't mean you don't have to manage what you eat. You do. So portion size was the next thing I had to work on—and I'm still working on it even now. To get things under control, I started to eat more slowly and began to put less on my plate. I'm finding that the more I do these things, the more they become natural parts of my life.

To get my body moving, I began speedwalking and doing a little light jogging. Then I got lazy and stopped, and had to start up again. It's been a struggle, but I'm doing it.

It took me a year to lose the first 15 pounds, and I stayed at 240 for a long time, almost a year. I'll be honest, part of me considered turning to a fad diet. But I didn't want to get sick. Finally I began to understand that eating healthfully simply had to be my way of life. I never really got that before. Once I could see that the changes I'd made were forever, I was able to move forward. That's when I really pushed myself into gear, committing myself to eating properly and working out. I lost another 30 pounds in seven months. Since then I've shed 10 more pounds and I'm still losing little by little. I'd like to drop 25 more pounds. I went from a size 22 to a size 16, and I want to get to a 14. I'd be happy at a 14. I don't want to be skinny. I want to be healthy.

I'm proud of what I've accomplished thus far. I'm so happy that God has graced me to help stop me from continuing on that downward path. That's what it was. Obesity is killing black women. We need to eat better. We need to make some conscious choices. People say, "Well, my grandmother ate that way and she lived to be 80." That may be true, but she was also probably on her knees scrubbing floors or doing some other hard physical work. We're sitting behind desks and dying at age 40.

Even though I'm not yet at the weight I'd like to be, I can honestly tell you that I feel free. I will never "diet" again. The changes I've made will last me a lifetime because I realize what's at risk and I understand what I need to do. There's a verse in the Bible that reads, "My people perish because of lack of knowledge." We have to be knowledgeable about nutrition and health. Don't worry so much about weight; focus on health.

CHAPTER 7

⚜

It's a Family Thing

When a sister makes up her mind to lose weight, she has much more to consider than how many pounds to drop. Starting a weight-loss program is never a solitary pursuit, especially not for black women. You may be the one trying to shed pounds, but you know everybody's going to have to put in their two cents.

First up: your man. We come from a culture that favors curvaceous women, and your husband or boyfriend may not want you to peel off too many pounds, if any at all. But you know that you need to do so in order to improve your health. Some brothers may even be afraid that if you lose the weight, they might lose you. Of course it sounds ridiculous to you—you love the brother, and fitting into a smaller dress size isn't going to change that. But many men see it differently. The slimmer you get, the more nervous and afraid they become. Truth be told, getting fit can have a big impact on your love relationships.

You want your honey to be happy, but you also want to do what's best for you. Putting your health first without alienating the man in your life is a very real concern for many black women. For single sisters, the same holds true. You know there are lots of brothers out there who like voluptuous women, and that very thought may be in the back of your mind as you begin our program and hit the dating scene, too. Just know this: If you don't have your health, you won't have much of anything else.

Next up: your family. You want to toss out the chips and cookies that tempt your tongue, but your children ain't having it. How many times can you hear, "But Ma!" before you give in? You want to cook more chicken and fish, and less red meat. But your husband is a hard-core steak-and-potatoes man. Lord knows, when it comes to losing weight, family is often the toughest obstacle sisters face. Your husband and children want to eat the foods they've always eaten, and the constant nagging and whining is enough to drive any sane sister crazy.

You can understand where they're coming from, though. They love your famous barbecue ribs. Or is it your fried chicken? Can't forget about that cobbler. Whatever your specialty, your family doesn't want you to stop making it. But you know you have to cut back on those foods in order to lose weight. Therein lies the problem: how to offer your family foods they will accept and enjoy at the same time that you are trying to get in shape. You don't want to deny them favorite dishes, but you also don't want to deny yourself a fit body.

Then there's the time-management issue. Your goal is to squeeze in a good workout several times a week, but between your job, your husband's work, your kids' schedules, and all sorts of other commitments, who has time? So you struggle to fit it in. Some weeks you're successful. Other weeks . . . well, let's not even go there.

Last up: everybody else. As much as your friends and relatives cheer your efforts to lose weight, there's bound to be one or two who jump on your last nerve. You know the type—fake smile plastered on her face, telling you how much thinner you look and how happy she is for you, all the while offering you a slice of pie and a "Oh, one piece won't hurt." Or the other types who only have nice things to say to your face, but the minute you turn your back they're crowing about how you'll never lose the weight.

Saboteurs, plain and simple. These are the people who, for whatever reason—jealousy perhaps?—don't want to see you succeed.

On the flip-side of saboteurs are the food police—family and friends who are "only trying to help." Don't reach for a second helping or you're going to hear about it. "Now girl, you know you don't need that!" Or "I thought you were trying to lose weight." Or "Are you sure you can have that on your diet?" Meanwhile, you know very well what you can have and how much. As you sit there, stunned, thinking *No she didn't say that to me,* the food police have accomplished their goal—undermining your efforts in a lame attempt to "help."

What a Wonderful World It Would Be

By now, you may be wishing you could block out the rest of the world and simply concentrate on yourself. It would be wonderful if you could scrap the interference and just do what you need to do to lose weight, wouldn't it? Eat healthy foods without someone constantly getting in your ear about it. Work out on a regular basis without having to accommodate three or four other people's schedules. Go about every day with ease, living your life in an active, healthy, invigorated way without anybody sticking their nose into your business. Ahh yes, it would be nice. But we can't live our lives with tunnel vision. You can't block out the rest of the world as you journey toward a healthier, fitter body. Nor should you waste time arguing, fighting, or bending over backward to please others. You have to strike a balance: Do what's best for you while keeping everything else harmonious. You want your mantra to be "It's all good." And you want to mean it. So the question is, how do you pull it off? By bringing everyone into the fold. Make your weight loss a family thing. The more involved they are, the better off you'll all be. Don't stop at your man and your kids. Open up your arms and your soul to all your friends, your siblings, your parents, your relatives. Let them in on what you are trying to accomplish, how important it is to you, and why you need their love and support. And make sure they truly understand that last part, because support is a whole lot different than butting in. Remember, we are a group-oriented people. Use that cultural gift to your advantage and you will find your journey much more pleasant and easy to navigate.

Taking Care of Number One

Just because our community tells us it's okay to be "thick," that doesn't mean we have to follow suit. You know the risks of carrying around too many pounds. Need a refresher course? Then read chapter 2 again. Chances are, you've seen the effects of overweight and obesity first hand in your own family. Genetics do play a part in all of this. Studies indicate that obesity is hereditary, so many of us are predisposed to heaviness. Having overweight parents may stack the odds against you, but you don't have to accept your family photos as destiny. Nor do you have to accept the desires of others. It's all about you, girl. You come first.

As much as you want to appeal to your husband, boyfriend, or the men you date, the bottom line is that you can't worry so much about what other folks think. You have to focus on your own health. Besides, you may be worrying for nothing. Your man says he doesn't want you to lose your curves. Well, guess what? You don't have to. Who says you have to be super-skinny to be healthy? You're not on the big screen. There's no camera around to add 10 pounds. That stick-figure stuff may play in Hollywood, but here in the real world many waif-thin women are far less healthy than their heavier counterparts. How is that possible? Because the numbers on the scale don't determine the fitness of your body. The percentage of fat you carry around is the real key.

When we meet with sister-patients, these are the two issues we always address. We talk with them about black folks' perception of body image, and try to get them to see that it's not about what others think. It's about how they feel, how their bodies function, how healthy they are. Then we tell them about BMI—body-mass index. BMI is a method of assessing your weight and your risk for weight-related health problems. For years, people relied on the old Metropolitan Life Insurance Company's height/weight charts, which were based on body-frame size, to determine if they were too fat. But BMI is a better measurement because instead of simply looking at body weight, BMI factors in your body-fat. What's the big deal about that? Well, for one thing, the amount of body-fat you have, and its location on your physique, are better predictors of health risk than how much you weigh.

Say a sister diets likes mad, but she never exercises. She'd much rather plop on the couch night after night rather than hit the gym. Her rationale? "My diet is working; the pounds are coming off. So why should I bother working out?" What sistergirl doesn't realize is that her constant dieting and chronic inactivity can lead to an unhealthy amount of body fat. When she steps on the scale and sees the numbers going down, she believes she's succeeding. She's losing weight all right, but it's lean muscle tissue, not fat. She's getting rid of the very thing she should be holding on to. On the other side of the coin is the muscular, fit sister who would easily be labeled overweight according to the old height/weight charts. When she steps on the scale, she may weigh more than the diets-like-crazy-and-never-moves-her-butt sister. But there's a big difference. The muscular sister is not over-fat, and therefore faces considerably less risk of weight-related health problems. The reason she may weigh more is because muscle is heavier than fat. But despite what the scale says, the muscular sister is far more healthy.

So don't let the numbers on the scale fool you. Use them as a guide, but pay attention to your BMI too. Keep in mind, though, that BMI is not a perfect tool. The muscular, fit sister could just as easily be categorized as overweight according to BMI figures too, even though she's not fat. And it would be precisely because she has more lean muscle tissue—it weighs more, so she weighs more.

The only way to truly find out how much of your body is fat and how much is muscle is with such body-composition measurement tools as skinfold calipers, an underwater weighing test, or a magnetic resonance imaging scan. However, you need a professional to administer these tests. So until there is a tool of self-measurement that takes all factors into precise account, we want you to be realistic about your BMI reading. For years, a BMI of 27 or more was considered the point at which a person could be classified as overweight. Then, in the summer of 1998, the National Institutes of Health released new BMI guidelines with 25 as the too-fat cutoff point. All of a sudden, people who thought they were at perfectly healthy weights were deemed overweight, and even obese. Different experts interpret BMI figures in different ways. Some agree with the new 25 cutoff; others don't. Perhaps there is a need for closer scrutiny. We certainly have heard from scores of African-American women who say that the charts don't fit them—that the guidelines are too stringent for black women. That's why we put the focus of our message squarely on the issue of health risk, and so should you.

To figure out your BMI, multiply your weight in pounds by 703.

WHAT'S YOUR BODY MASS INDEX?

BMI	19	20	21	22	23	24	25	26	27	28	29	30	35	40
Height						Weight in Pounds								
5'0"	97	102	107	112	118	123	128	133	138	143	148	153	179	204
5'1"	100	106	111	116	122	127	132	137	143	148	153	158	185	211
5'2"	104	109	115	120	126	131	136	142	147	153	158	164	191	218
5'3"	107	113	118	124	130	135	141	146	152	158	163	169	197	225
5'4"	110	116	122	128	134	140	145	151	157	163	169	174	204	232
5'5"	114	120	126	132	138	144	150	156	162	168	174	180	210	240
5'6"	118	124	130	136	142	148	155	161	167	173	179	186	216	247
5'7"	121	127	134	140	146	153	159	166	172	178	185	191	223	255
5'8"	125	131	138	144	151	158	164	171	177	184	190	197	230	262
5'9"	128	135	142	149	155	162	169	176	182	189	196	203	236	270
5'10"	132	139	146	153	160	167	174	181	188	195	202	207	243	278
5'11"	136	143	150	157	165	172	179	186	193	200	208	215	250	286

Chart courtesy of the National Institutes of Health.

Divide the answer by your height in inches. Divide that result by your height in inches again. Don't feel like fooling with all of that math? Then just locate your height and weight on the chart on page 131.

To find out your risk level, take a look at our suggested guidelines, which we feel are more realistic:

Your BMI	Your Health Risk
20–25	very low risk
26–30	low risk
31–35	moderate risk
36–40	high risk
40+	very high risk

Once you start working out and eating well, the fat will come off. In its place: calorie-burning muscle. You'll still have those sexy curves your man likes (you may even have more, thanks to your newly toned and well-defined body) but now you'll be stronger, fitter, and less prone to hypertension, diabetes, heart disease, and the myriad of other diseases connected with obesity.

Remember, a healthy lifestyle must be first and foremost in your life. If your man is the type who wants you to stay just the way you are, you may not be able to change his mindset overnight. After all, he comes from the same culture you do—the one that's told both of you for years that bigger is better. But if you can change your attitude, he can certainly change his.

Here's what you do: Sit him down and explain the risks you face by remaining overweight. You may want to have him read chapter two as well. Seeing the facts on paper opened your eyes. Perhaps it will open his, too.

We can't emphasize enough how important it is to put your health ahead of all else. No one can make this journey to wellness for you. No one but you can give you back control of your life. The power to achieve your goal truly comes from within. Understanding and support from the man you love will definitely make the going easier, but if it takes him awhile to give it, you know what you have to do. Reach down within yourself and find the mettle to keep going—to stick with your plan. Continue talking to him and educating him about your weight-loss goal. He'll come around. In the meantime, let your inner strength and resolve keep you on the right course. You can do it.

The Ties That Bind

Although the success of this fitness journey demands that you put yourself first, we know that you can't simply close your eyes to loved ones. Blinders don't work when it comes to family. They will just snatch them off and get in your face anyway. If family can't speak their minds, who can? Those kinship bonds and emotional ties to your husband, your children, and your relatives are an important and everlasting part of your life. And putting your own needs ahead of everyone else can often seem selfish. Girlfriend, we're here to tell you it's not. Losing excess weight and improving your health is never a selfish pursuit.

First of all, doing so will extend your life expectancy, which means you'll be around longer for your loved ones. Second, by striving to become fit, you will be a positive role model for your children, especially your daughters. A study sponsored by the National Heart, Lung and Blood Institute in the 1980s showed a correlation between overweight in black teenage girls and overweight in their mothers. When you embark on a wellness plan, your daughter is apt to follow suit. Research shows that black girls get much of their information about weight control from family members. What's more, a 1990 study published in the journal *Pediatrics* found that adolescent African-American girls who participated in a weight-loss program were more likely to be successful when their mothers participated too. It's obvious that Mama wields a lot of influence. As you can see, what may have seemed like a selfish pursuit to you a few minutes ago will have a very positive impact on your family.

Think about all of the other wonderful benefits you stand to gain as you lose.

- You'll reduce your risk of obesity-related diseases.
- You'll improve your blood pressure.
- You'll be stronger.
- You'll boost your self-esteem, confidence, as well as your self-appreciation.
- Your inner beauty will shine through because you'll know you're successfully going after your goal.
- You'll discover a desire to do new things you may have been afraid to try before.
- You'll have a ton of energy.
- You'll feel better than you have in years.
- You'll develop a whole new attitude.

So go ahead. Be "selfish" about your health. It's the most loving and giving thing you can do for your family.

It's a Family Affair

Nothing helps us succeed in life like support from loved ones. When someone's in your corner, telling you you can do it, there's no stopping you. Obstacles be damned. When you have a strong rooting section, you find a way past those roadblocks. You go around them, or over them, or under them, or just barrel right through them. This journey you're embarking on cries out for that kind of support. Yes, you can reach your goal-weight range on your own. You're a strong black woman who is committed to taking charge of her health and her life. If need be, we know you can go it alone—successfully changing your eating and exercise habits for the better. But flying solo will only make your journey more difficult and your path more strewn with roadblocks. Relying on yourself for encouragement and motivation is certainly important—you are your number one cheerleader, after all—but tapping your inner reserve over and over again can also be draining. Having a support system in place, however, gives you another reserve to fall back on.

One of your support systems is your sister circle. Your girls have got your back so you know you can count on them whenever willpower starts to wane. Your other support system should be your immediate family—your husband and your children. (You single sisters can reach out to your siblings, parents, tight friends, or anyone who is very close to you, whom you see regularly.) Knowing that loved ones are behind you as you strive to get fit can help you succeed. Losing weight isn't easy. It takes commitment, hard work, and a whole new attitude. Imagine how tough it's going to be if you change your way of thinking and no one else in the household does. No one's saying they have to do everything you do, right down to the last bicep curl. (Although if your husband needs to shed a few pounds and opts to shape up with you, all the better.) We're talking about emotional support—understanding your goals, encouraging your efforts, not doing anything to hinder your progress, helping you stay on track, being accommodating to your healthier lifestyle. Not only will family support increase your odds of losing the weight, it will also bring you all closer.

You will all be sharing in a common goal—namely, improving your health—which can only strengthen your family's bond. As we've said before, gaining their support may not happen overnight. But we want you to see how beneficial and crucial it is for you. As you attempt to bring your loved ones into the fold, you may get fed up if they don't get with the program right away. The simple fact is, your husband and kids may not be open to your healthier lifestyle, even though you assure them that it won't mean a drastic change in their way of life, in the way *they* eat or what *they* do. You may tell them again and again that this is about *you* changing *your* life—with their help. But, unfortunately, they may not believe it. That's when those roadblocks start going up: They ask for foods you're trying to cut back on or avoid, and even bring foods home that you just can't resist. Meanwhile, you're left wondering why they're trying to make it harder for you. "Don't they know how tough this is for me?" you ask yourself. Listen sisterfriend, here's where their heads are at: They probably think they will have to give up all of the foods they love, or that you will constantly nag them about how they're not getting enough exercise or that they're eating too much junk. And at times, that latter prediction will come true. Some of us do get a bit overzealous when we are attempting to lose weight. We want everyone we care about to be the best they can be, too. Okay, let's admit it, sometimes we simply nag out of frustration. This is hard work and it can be tough to see others lounging around eating like pigs while we're sweating our tails off and trying to alter the way we think about food.

So you have to make a promise to your family that you will try to keep your inner zealot and inner nag under control, and they have to promise to try to give you the support you need. If you can all agree to at least try, you'll be taking a big step. In a few short weeks you'll all see how easy it is to uphold those promises. You'll be getting closer, and you'll feel like you are in this thing together. Before you know it, you all won't be "trying" to hold up your ends of the bargain, you'll simply be doing it.

Getting to that point, however, takes planning. How are you going to bring all of this up with your husband and children? What will you say? How can you get them involved? What can you do to convince them to help you? You know and we know that it's difficult to change someone's attitude, beliefs, or habits. The change *can* occur, but it's going to require motivation, strategic planning, faith, and determination on your part. Most of all, you're going to need to be in an "I Can Do This" state of mind.

Can I Talk to Y'all for a Minute?

The first step toward gaining your family's support is to have a family meeting right from the start. Involving them at the beginning of your journey sends the message that they are important to you and to your success. Gather your husband and children in the living room, kitchen, wherever you all feel most comfortable. Now is the time for complete and total honesty. (Your husband will have already heard this, but he can hear it again.) Tell them, point blank, that you are going to lose weight, and tell them why. Be blunt. Don't pull any punches about the risks to your health. Lay it all out on the table: high blood pressure, diabetes, heart disease, and all of the other problems that are linked to obesity. If your children are young, you may have to break it down in terms they can understand: "Mommy has made up her mind to lose weight because it will help keep me from getting sick" or something along those lines. Older kids and teenagers can be given more specific details. We're not talking scare tactics here, just straightforward, clear information. Then tell your family that you're going to need their help in order to get healthy. Explain what you have learned about eating healthfully and how you plan to change the way you eat. Let them know that the Soul Food Pyramid you will be using as your guide leaves plenty of room for the down-home foods they enjoy so much, and that favorite dishes will still find their way to the table on a regular basis. There's no need to spill all of your secrets, however. Why tell them exactly how you plan to substitute certain foods or alter your recipes? Keep the exact details to yourself. They'll never know the difference, not with the healthy soul recipes and cooking strategies we give you in these pages. Trust us, your family will be too busy smacking their lips over your good cooking.

Next, tell you family about your exercise routine. Let them know your workout schedule and fill them in on your sister circle too. Tell them what the sister circle is, what it's all about, and how it will function. Last but not least, ask your husband and your kids to have faith in you as you begin your journey to wellness and to accept your progress no matter how small it is. Five or ten pounds may not seem like a big deal to others, but it's a major victory for you. When loved ones acknowledge these milestones, it strengthens your conviction to keep going. Make sure they know that.

Once your family sees that you are serious about improving your health, they'll be more inclined to give you the support you need.

Family + Fitness = Fun

You know you're more apt to stick to your exercise plan when you have someone sweating it out right alongside you. That's one of the reasons for your sister circle. Every "Come on girl, you can do it" keeps you moving when you feel like falling out. Why stop with your sisterfriends? Get your husband and kids into the act. They don't have to do your workout routine with you, but they can be physically active with you. Consider the benefits: You'll squeeze in extra exercise during the week, your husband and kids will reap their own health rewards (getting your kids into the habit of being physically active will be the start of a fitness mindset that can last a lifetime), and it will give all of you a chance to spend more time together—an especially nice bonus given the hectic pace of most sisters' lives these days.

Here's one easy way to exercise with your family: Take walks together after dinner. A walk through the neighborhood not only gives you the opportunity for added exercise, it also gives you a chance to catch up on one another's day and to say "hey" to your neighbors who may be sitting out on the porch or tending their lawns. Why not designate certain evenings of the week as family walk nights, and head outdoors while it's still light?

Another idea: Get outside on the weekends and play games together. Your backyard will do fine—or head on down to a nearby park. Play basketball, softball, volleyball, touch football, soccer, whatever is fun for all of you. Take a bike ride together. Play freeze tag. Whatever your kids would normally do for fun, join in with your husband. If your children balk at the idea of playing with Moms and Pops, then make it a challenge. The "old folks" versus the "young'uns." Odds are, they'll take that bet, if only to try to show you up. Who cares who wins? The point is to do something active together. You'll be inching closer and closer to your goal because of all the extra exercise. Your family will get in more fun quality time together. And, best of all, you'll be making them a part of your fitness journey—whether they realize it or not.

Is your husband tied up at work or stuck with a prior obligation? You don't have to wait for him to have fun with your kids. You can do any of these activities with them by yourself. Then, when it's time for a little togetherness with your man, call the babysitter and plan a sweaty night for two. (Not that kind of sweat, girl! Y'all can save that for later. Hmm. Come to think of it, that is a good way to burn up some calories!) Remember when we told you to hit the clubs with your sister circle for exercise? Well, do the same thing with your husband. When's the last time the two of you got all hot and bothered on the dance floor? It's time to do it again, girlfriend.

Are you starting to see how easy it is to get your family involved in your fitness plans? As long as your body's moving and your heart's pumping, it counts as exercise. Squeeze some of these extra activities in a few times every week and you'll reach your weight-loss goal faster than you think.

Come On and Eat

Food. Here's where you're most likely to meet up with some resistance from the family. No matter how many times you tell them that your cooking will taste good, they are going to have something to say. They know you are eating more healthfully, which means you are cooking more healthfully, so of course they think that means bland food that tastes terrible. What to do? Keep some things secret.

Small changes in preparation—say, using low-fat milk and low-fat cheese instead of the more calorie- and fat-laden originals—won't have a strong effect on the taste. Chances are your family won't even know you've made a change. If they don't mention anything, why should you? Take spaghetti and meatballs. If it's one of your kids' favorites (and yours, too), try making the meatballs with ground turkey instead of ground beef, but don't tell anyone about the switch. Now sit back and check out the reaction. We'll bet there won't be one, other than "This is good, Ma."

Now, we don't want to seem as if we are advocating out-and-out lying. We told you to be honest with your family at your family meeting, and we meant it. But if you have the type of husband and the type of children who just can't live without certain dishes, why set the stage for a big hassle? Keep quiet and go on about the business of healthy cooking.

That said, we do believe you should include your family in meal preparation and planning. Bring them into the kitchen to help fix some of the meals. Get everybody involved in the peripheral tasks—chopping, mixing, tossing. Remember, the chef doesn't want all of her healthy secrets getting out; that's why you only let them handle certain tasks. Don't give them the opportunity to turn their noses up at a dish before even tasting it. Whatever job they handle in the kitchen, the final result will be a more accepting family. When your husband and kids have a hand, literally, in preparing healthy meals, they will be more likely to give each dish the thumbs-up. As for meal planning, ask them what favorite foods they'd like to have each week. This will make grocery shopping easier since you will know what meals you'll be preparing beforehand and what food substitutions and spices will be required. Then, when you set the table and dish up their favorites, they will be happy that they didn't have to give them up just because you're trying to lose weight. All the while, you will have fixed the food in a healthier way, so you can sit down and enjoy it alongside everyone else.

Okay, let's be quite real for a moment. There are some foods that are going to have to go. And no amount of nagging and whining should sway you. Ice cream, potato chips, cookies, barbecue skins, fatty cold cuts, and all of those other "gonna-go-right-to-your-hips" foods should get tossed out. If your family gives you lip, tell them that you're willing to brainstorm replacements. Ice cream is out, but ice milk or frozen yogurt is all right. Potato chips—forget it. Air-popped popcorn and pretzels—perfect. Make trade-offs that will work for you and your family. Remember, this is about you and your health. So although you may have to bend on some issues—like giving your family time to adjust to your new way of doing things—you cannot compromise when it comes to temptation. If you know you are likely to pig out on certain unhealthy foods—your trigger foods—don't keep them in the house, period. Your family will get used to this change in time, especially if there are other "Mama-approved" snacks in the kitchen to munch on.

When you are the only person in the household who's eating healthfully in order to lose weight, it can be difficult. That's a given. You have to satisfy everyone's taste buds in order to keep the peace. While you can't force your weight-loss plan on others (except for those trigger foods—we mean it when we say keep 'em out of the house), you can encourage your family to be proactive and teach them how to practice healthy lifestyle changes. With time and patience you can get your husband and children to adapt to at least some of the changes. You have to decide how far you're willing to bend without jeopardizing your own goals. Keep reminding yourself that this journey is about your health. It's a balancing act, to be sure, but we know you can make it work. Continue talking to your family; keep reminding them of your goals and the reason for your journey. Don't worry about sounding like a broken record. Once you've shed the pounds, it really won't matter how much talking and convincing you had to do to get there, will it? You will have succeeded and, in the end, that's all that matters.

Stop the Sabotage

No matter how much support you get from your husband, children, and even your friends and extended family, sooner or later you are going to run across one of the C.A.D.S.—commentators, agitators, dictators, and spectators. They are the saboteurs and food police we told you about earlier: the ones who may be jealous of your resolve or of your progress, the ones who may have their own weight problems and can't seem to get a handle on them, the ones who may not have the love and support in their lives that you do. There are any number of reasons that would drive C.A.D.S. to give you a hard time. But you know what? There's no use wasting your time trying to figure out their every motive. What you should do instead is find a way to deal. Don't let anyone—not friends, relatives, or colleagues—get in the way of your progress. Just think of the C.A.D.S. as another roadblock to bust through. No need to break out the steamroller. There are ways to handle these people which don't require getting down and dirty. First of all, know exactly who you're dealing with:

Commentators—These people get in your face with untruths and unsolicited, nonfactual opinions. They will spout off about the calories in that biscuit, chicken, or whatever else you're about to eat, and the information will be wrong. They'll comment on your workout, advising you on what you *should* be doing, and the information will be wrong. Do you see a pattern emerging here? Commentators think they know everything—or at least more than you do—and their information will be . . . well, you know. When you hit 'em with the facts, do they back down? Please! Their tongues keep right on wagging. There's just no arguing with these people.

Agitators—These are the folks who are always looking to start something. Remember back in school there was always one girl off on the sidelines talking out of both sides of her mouth, egging people on until a fight broke out? Back in the day, we called that girl an instigator. Today, with agitators, it's the same difference. They egg you on until you break out the food. Think of them as the hard-core saboteurs. They're the ones offering you foods they know you can't resist. They're the pesky mosquitoes in your ear, buzzing about how "one piece won't hurt" until you give in. Afterward, you feel guilty and wish you had swatted them away. You need strong willpower when these people are around.

Dictators—They say they want to help, but what they really want to do is run your life. These folks are the food police, always trying to tell you how to eat. They take things a step farther than the commentators, because not only will dictators put in their two cents, they'll get downright physical with you. A dictator will take a piece of food right off your plate or out of your hand. We're not kidding. If they see you heading for an item on the buffet table that they think is no good for you, they'll walk over and remove the platter. We're talking serious nerve here. Dictators like to run their mouths, and they'll back it up, too.

Spectators—These people are always looking for an opportunity to see you fail. They keep a sharp eye peeled for any slip-ups, and then they let you and everybody else hear about it. You feel like you have to be on your best behavior when you're around a spectator—and even when you're not. If they spy you pulling out of the McDonald's drive-through when you're supposed to be at the gym, girl, don't you know half the town is going to know it. Whatever the situation, if a spectator sees you fall off the wagon, phones will be ringing. "I told you she wouldn't be able to stay on a diet." "I told you she'd stop going to the gym." "I told you she wasn't going to lose that weight." Spectators watch you like a hawk, and the minute you mess up they swoop down for all the juicy details.

So how do you shut up the C.A.D.S.? Rather than telling someone off (you'll just waste breath and energy), try reasoning with them calmly and getting them to see how much their comments and actions undermine your efforts. Sometimes this approach works. Some people will understand where you're coming from and back off; some may even offer you genuine support once you open their eyes to their destructive behavior. But there will always be those knuckleheaded folks who just won't get it. No matter how much you talk to them, they won't change. And as we've said, you can't waste your time arguing and pleading with people; it will only distract you from your ultimate goal.

If some of these people don't want to hear what you're trying to say, then do the same to them. It will be difficult at first; letting negativity roll off your back isn't easy for anyone. It hurts. But sister, think about the alternative: constantly being on the defensive, always feeling judged. Why put up with that? Our advice is to let hurtful, negative, sabotage-loaded comments go in one ear and out the other. So-called friends, relatives, and colleagues don't want to be supportive? Then bump 'em. Don't let them hold you back. Remind yourself that there are many folks who do support you, who do want to see you succeed, especially your sister circle. Turn to your sister circle if you have a run-in with one of the C.A.D.S. and need a bit of loving counterbalance. Rely on your inner strength too to tune out or walk away from those who try to pull you down. It's going to take inner strength to deflect the negativity, but we're confident you can do it.

You may be surprised by the result. Sometimes when C.A.D.S. see that their actions can't faze you or get a rise out of you, they'll stop. They may even treat you with newfound respect, because they will know that you're serious about getting fit, and that you're not going to let them or anyone else stop you. Who knows? One day they may come to you for advice and support if they start a fitness plan. Now wouldn't that be an ironic turn of events?

Remember, It's All About You

Now that you know how to cope with the outside world—family, friends, relatives—it's time to do some inner work. Making your fitness journey a family affair is sure to aid in your success, but you can't ever forget that all of this—eating well, working out regularly, staying focused and committed—starts and ends with you. You are accountable to yourself alone. Sometimes the outside world is going to make the journey tough on you. Sometimes you'll make it tough on yourself. There will be times when you struggle with your own mind, but you have to maintain a strong heart, sister. Keep thinking about how much better your life will be once you've shed those pounds. Keep that positive inner dialogue going. Don't let negative inner thoughts deter you; don't let moments of weakness set you back; don't beat yourself up if you stumble. Just pick yourself up and take another step, and another, and another. We know you have a jumble of doubts swimming in your head. "Can I do this? Will I succeed?" Focus on the goal. Here are a few tips, strategies, and words of advice to help you stay on-point.

- Love yourself.
- Reaffirm your personal goals each and every day.
- Take a hard look at your values, beliefs, and self-esteem. What motivates you? Are there issues in your life that might hold you back from success? Try to deal with them and move on.
- Keep your sights set on achieving good health. Don't categorize what you are doing as simply "dieting."

- Do you have a tendency to be a perfectionist? Let it go. That way of thinking is a sure-fire formula for failure. No one is perfect. All we can ask of ourselves is to try our best.
- Instill a sense of purpose and positivity into your own life and it will impact others. Remember, positivity is contagious.
- Make lifestyle changes gradually. Don't try to do everything at once.
- Find healthful foods you enjoy that can be used as snacks. Reach for those first when you get a craving to munch on something.
- Drink plenty of H_2O every day. Add lime or lemon to your water to make it more zesty, refreshing, and satisfying.
- Keep boredom at bay. We often turn to food when we have nothing to do. Add enjoyable, planned activities to your schedule if this sounds like you.
- Keep a food diary. Jot down everything that goes in your mouth. Be sure also to write how you felt as you ate and what motivated you to eat.
- Reward yourself when you reach a milestone—a beautiful new scarf, a hot CD, the latest bestseller, a professional manicure, have your man give you a massage—anything other than food that will bring you pleasure. Or simply call a good friend and tell her about your fitness achievement. Let her happiness for you and her encouragement be your reward.
- Go through your cupboards and give them a good purging. Read every label and ask yourself if the item fits in with your new and improved way of eating. Donate those products that don't to a shelter—the feeling you'll get from helping others is sure to keep you on a positive tip. Replace the donated items with healthier choices.
- Don't allow yourself to become chained to the scale.
- Keep in mind that even the smallest step is a major achievement.

- No success comes without some failure along the way. Whenever you falter, try to learn from it and keep on stepping.
- Take a few moments every day to reflect on your blessings.
- Trust in your faith. No matter what ups and downs you face on this journey and in life, your faith will always be there to see you through.

Sister to Sister
✗◇✗◇✗◇✗◇✗

Julia Weaver, a thirty-five-year-old assistant buyer from
  Stone Mountain, Georgia
Current weight: 146 pounds
Amount lost: 105 pounds

To this day I don't know why I started gaining weight. I've always been a very positive person and an extremely happy person. So it wasn't as if I was eating for comfort or to feel better. But I was eating. And eating and eating. The most I'd ever weighed was 120 pounds, but after I got married I started gaining. Over the years I've tried exercising and even starving myself, but nothing worked. I was tired, irritable, and worried about my health. And one of my close relatives didn't help matters.

She was probably the worst person for me to be around at the time. She always made comments about my weight. One time she said, "I don't know what we're going to do with you. You have such a beautiful face but you have ruined your body. You're going to be 400 pounds before you know it." My two children were with me at the time and I was so hurt by her comment. I just said to her, "Don't go there." What was I going to say? She's my elder and I have to respect her. Plus my children were standing there listening to my response. Afterward, I got in my truck with tears streaming down my face. The person who was the closest to me was hurting me the most. I suppose she said those things because she thought it was going to help me. But it didn't. When I got home following that incident, I talked to my husband about it, and then I ate some ice cream. Hmm. It seems I was using food to comfort myself after all. I guess eating was my way to get back at her.

She is extremely attractive and fashion-forward. She used to model. I know she was embarrassed by me, and that was probably the hardest thing I had to come to grips with.

My husband might make a few comments about my weight when we had a fuss, but nowhere near as much as this particular relative. He tried to encourage me to go to the gym or go walking and my response was, "I don't want to go." Whenever he tried to encourage me, I took it as a negative and blew him off.

Finally something in me made me realize that I had to try and shed some weight. I thought about how I felt. I thought about what the weight could do to my health. I thought about my two children and how I wanted to be around for them. I guess I thought about a lot of things. The point is, I finally went to the doctor and had a full physical. I started walking the next day. I could only do ten minutes at first because I'd get so tired. But I slowly worked up to 35 minutes every day—which is what I still do today. After I'd shed some pounds, I started jumping rope, too. I roller-skate every Friday night now as well and just lead a more active life.

To improve my eating, I began keeping track of fat grams and calories, stopped eating fried foods and drinking soda, scaled way back on red meat, and drank at least 64 ounces of water a day. My big thing is chocolate, so what I'd do is have two little Tootsie Rolls and I was set. I discovered that that's all I needed to satisfy my chocolate craving. I stopped making excuses, too. I was working a lot, trying to take care of my family, always rushing here and there. I ate on the run, stopping at McDonald's for a burger and fries. I cut that out. Now I cook healthy, balanced meals for myself. If I make hamburgers for my kids and husband, I'll bake a chicken along with it for me to eat.

It was very hard in the beginning, but I kept at it. I lost 19 pounds the first month. Ten pounds the second month. Eight pounds the month after that. I hit a plateau after about six months. I wasn't losing anything. Of course, I started thinking that I couldn't do it anymore. But I looked in the mirror and said to myself, "You know what, girl-friend? You have gotten this far. You can make it." I guess I'd gotten to the point where I finally realized that I had to do this for myself and no one else—not my friends, not my husband, no one. I know that if you try to lose the weight for another person you'll never keep it off. If you do it for yourself, you'll be able to do anything.

Since I've lost the weight, that close relative I mentioned before has been more accepting of me. I've had to let go of the hurt she caused me, because life is too short. However, I still want to sit down with her and talk to her about how her comments made me feel. I think that's something I have to do. The most important thing, though, is that I'm healthy. I have a four-year-old and an eight-year-old, and I didn't want to wake up one day with heart problems caused by being overweight. I want to be here to enjoy their lives.

Since I dropped over 100 pounds, people are always saying to me, "My gosh, look how much you've lost!" Sometimes they don't even know who I am. I hadn't seen my godmother in nearly a year and I saw her at a friend's birthday party. She walked in and I said, "Hey." My god-mother looked at me then asked someone, "Who is that?"

She didn't recognize me because I'd gone from a size 24 to a size 10.

People may say, "Oh girl, you look good." But it's not about that. It's about how I feel. And I feel great. When you are finally able to understand that the external is just the packaging and the internal is what's truly important, it's a beautiful experience.

CHAPTER 8

⋈

Ain't No Stopping You Now

Y*ou go, girl!* Won't be long before you're hearing that left and right. You're on your way, sisterfriend. You're doing it. You're eating right, cooking up some mouth-watering—and healthy—soul food. You're exercising on a regular basis, moving that body, and working up a serious sweat. Your sister circle is in full swing, offering you the kind of support you need to reach your goal. Before you know it, family and friends will be commenting on how much slimmer you look. Folks you haven't seen in a while will say, "Girl, you look good. Have you lost some weight?" You'll flash them a big grin because you'll know you've done much more than that. You will have taken control of your life. Others may only see your newly sleek physique, but you'll know the real benefits: better health and a longer life.

Getting to that point is only half the battle, though. Once there, you will have to stay there. Many sisters can tell you story after story about how they lost weight and then put it right back on. Just as you have to be mentally and spiritually ready to start losing the pounds, so it is when you are trying to keep them off. This journey you've embarked upon is a life-long commitment. It takes work to shed the weight—you know that. So it makes sense that it will take more work to maintain the loss. We're not trying to discourage you. Just the opposite. We want you to be prepared for what's ahead. Anyone who tells you that losing weight and keeping it off is a breeze is lying to your face. (If it was that easy, we'd all be in great shape.) The real deal is that this requires effort. But once you truly commit to it, something clicks in your head. You "get it." You understand what it is you need to do to succeed. The process is sort of like having an awakening or an epiphany. All of a sudden everything makes sense, and you give yourself over to the journey. You're there, girlfriend. You've had that awakening. So keep it going.

Turning the Corner

As you journey toward fitness, you are going to hit a few bumps in the road. We've already told you how to handle them, so when they crop up we have no doubt that you'll find a way past them and continue on. Once you've lost the weight, you will look back at those obstacles and stumbling blocks and congratulate yourself for staying focused and moving forward. You made a promise to yourself and you kept it. You achieved what so many other black women struggle to achieve every day. Do you know what that says about you? You have determination, courage, faith, strength, and a powerful sense of commitment. Your self-esteem is going to be sky-high when you reach your goal. Enjoy the feeling; hold on to it. But don't rest on your laurels. While you are on that "I did it" cloud, refocus attention toward your new commitment: keeping the weight off.

You've turned the corner, and the new path on this continuing journey is one of maintenance. Before you begin the next phase, however, be sure to take care of some very important business. Let everyone who encouraged you know how grateful you are. Tell them how much their faith and support helped you along the way, and that you're going to need it even more as you proceed on this new path. When we struggle to accomplish something as important as improving our health, we definitely need the folks we love in our corner rooting us on. So take this opportunity to express your thanks.

Now, let's look to the future. Maintenance. What is it and how do you get some? Well, first of all, realize that it's a way of life. It's how you have to live every day once you've lost weight. Striving to get fit means making a lifestyle change, and maintenance is simply a continuation of the change.

For months you've altered the way you think about food, exercise, and the way you live your life. You eat differently now, and you're much more active. You have different priorities and a different mindset. If you expect to stay trimmed-down and healthy, you can't go back to your old ways. You have to really put your mind to continuing to eat healthfully and exercising regularly. Just because you've lost the weight doesn't mean that the changes you made in your life are over. Start backsliding again and again, and pretty soon you won't have to slide anymore—you'll be all the way back to where you started. The bottom line is that your new lifestyle has to be your only lifestyle.

Too often sisters who have lost weight try to wing it afterward. They think, "I've come this far, how hard can it be? I'll figure something out." Chances are, they didn't see losing the weight as a lifestyle change in the first place. They probably thought of it as a diet, plain and simple. Those sisters figured they'd lose the weight and once it was gone it would stay gone. Sorry, things don't work that way. Forget about the concept of "diet." That term is a failure trap. Instead, resolve to "do it." Now there's a positive, active, empowering phrase if we've ever heard one.

How are you going to get in shape? You're going to take the information we're giving you in these pages and come up with a plan of action. Guess what: It's the same with maintenance. You need a plan. Think of maintenance like driving a car. You have to do right by your ride to keep it running. Give it bad fuel, let it idle, and it will cut off on you. You have to do right by your body, too, if you want to keep it in good condition. Give it the wrong foods, don't keep it moving, and it will revert back to its old self.

When you're out on the highway, the signs ahead let you know where you're going, right? You navigate by those road signs. It's the same with weight maintenance. There are road signs on that path, too—indicators of where you're going. The trick is figuring out which ones will lead you in the wrong direction. That's why sisters who try to wing maintenance wind up backsliding rather than moving forward. They didn't heed the signs along the road. They didn't have a plan. You, however, know better.

Taming the Triggers

Keeping off the weight would be so much easier if maintenance really were like driving down the street. We could just look for the STOP sign and go the other way. Of course, it's not that simple. The signs you're looking for are more subtle. They come in the form of situations that can make you veer off track. Imagine you've dropped 20, 40, maybe 60 pounds and you're cruising along just fine. Then suddenly, BOOM! You're hit by something that sends your resolve into a tailspin. Next thing you know, you're tempted to chow down on fattening foods, or drink lots of high-calorie cocktails, or simply eat too much of everything. Before you can get your willpower in check, you're pigging out and telling yourself that there is no turning back. Soon, thoughts of your old habits start creeping into your head. You allow yourself to think about eating the way you used to and nixing the workouts that have become a part of your regular routine. Bottom line? You start thinking about giving up. All because of one incident, one situation that caught you sleeping and hit you full force. What was that something that knocked the resolve right out of you? A "trigger situation."

Trigger situations are the moments that test you, that make you doubt yourself, that have you doing double-takes, that tempt you to do the wrong thing. They could be birthday parties, Christmas festivities, Sunday dinners at Mama's house—any event that puts you and tons of food together and leaves you to fend for yourself. When we're faced with these trigger situations, we sometimes let temptation get the better of us because of the social setting. We're around other folks. Everyone's eating, drinking, and having a good time, and we don't want to be left out. Often the lure of food is harder to resist when we're in the company of others. People egg us on and we don't want to put a damper on the festivities, or we don't want to seem like the odd woman out. This one's munching on some fried chicken, that one's reaching for the Kahlúa, and we're just standing there looking. We want to have fun too. (Isn't it funny how so many of us associate food with fun?)

There are other times, though, when we overdo on the food because of stress, anger, sadness, anxiety, or any number of other powerful emotions. When you're feeling out of sorts and you're at some food-filled function, it's no wonder you grab the pigs-in-a-blanket rather than the crudité. Many of us have a tendency to use food as a coping mechanism, and a social setting simply puts added pressure on us to eat for comfort.

Sister, the world doesn't stop just because you're trying to keep off the weight—and it never will. No one is going to give up a bumping party to help you out. The question is, why should you sit home when there's a good time going on somewhere? Go ahead, take part. You've got to keep living too, girl. Remember when we told you that deprivation is out and moderation is in? Well, the same applies here. Don't hole up in the house and avoid get-togethers out of fear. You don't have to become a hermit to cope with trigger situations. What you need is a plan.

Every holiday celebration, party, family dinner, office function, catered conference, and the like is a tempting situation that can coerce you into eating more than you should. It's okay to indulge now and then—what the hell kind of life would it be otherwise?—but fall off the food wagon too many times and the wagon will leave you behind.

Different sisters have different trigger situations. For some, it might be celebrations involving sinfully delicious cake. For others, it could be parties where they can get their drink on. Still others may suffer from the "eyes are bigger than the stomach" syndrome at restaurants. (A six-page menu and a buffet table too? Watch out! If this sounds like you, go back to page 94 and review our "Dining Out the Right Way" tips.) What's your trigger? What type of situation puts your willpower to the test? Learn how to handle it, and maintaining your weight loss will be less of a challenge. Let's take a look at a few common triggers.

Trigger #1—Party Over Here!

Celebrate good times. Come on, let's celebrate. Black folks know how to have fun, don't we? The music's pumping, folks are dancing, seems like everyone's talking and laughing at once, and you know the food is flowing. We get so caught up in the festive mood that we don't even realize how much we've eaten. What the occasion is doesn't matter—it could be a birthday party for your sister, your girlfriend's wedding anniversary, your next-door neighbor's dinner party, your nephew's graduation blow-out, or just a family get-together. The point is, any time you are in a party atmosphere you run the risk of indulging a little too much.

There's no need to give up those good times. With a little forethought and strategic planning, you can keep your healthy habits in check even at the most tempting celebration. Next time you hit a party, put these tips into action.

- Don't skimp on food all day so that you can eat a lot that night. If you do, you're bound to be ravenous by the time you arrive at the party. And you know what that means! It's better to eat a normal breakfast and lunch, and have a light snack in the late afternoon or early evening. This way you won't make a beeline for the food the second you come through the door, and you'll be better able to select healthier foods when you are ready to eat.

- Check out what's available and stick to the healthier fare— for the most part. *Hmm. Fruit salad and the veggie platter, or buffalo wings and potato skins?* You know which ones are the better choices, but when everyone is reaching for the wings and skins, being good can be tough. So go ahead— have a bit, but don't go overboard. Fill up on the healthy offerings, and simply sample the "treats."

- *Uh-oh. There are no healthy offerings.* That wouldn't surprise us in the least. Lots of people just don't think about things like saturated fat, calories, cholesterol, and sodium when they're planning a party. That's why it pays to be prepared. Call your host ahead of time and ask what's on the menu. If every dish is a don't, then offer to bring something "for the party"—for instance, a mixed-greens salad with grilled chicken strips. Even if she says, "Oh girl, you don't have to do that," bring it anyway. No one has to know you're really bringing it for yourself.

Trigger #2—'Tis the Season . . . to Eat

The holidays are traditionally a time of gathering together as a family. And you know food plays a major role. Big, elaborate dinners at Christmas, Thanksgiving, and Easter. Backyard barbecues on the Fourth of July. Getting in the "spirits" on New Year's Eve. When a holiday rolls around, so do the calories. What is it about these special days that makes us want to overeat? Many of us view the holiday season as a license to chow down. We tell ourselves, "Well, it only comes around once a year." Never mind that we use that excuse five or six times a year.

The holidays also bring up lots of happy memories—memories we want to relive by following traditional celebrations of our past. So we continue the big dinners, the barbecues, and all the rest. Food ties us together during these special times of year. The downside, however, is that if you have lost weight, the holidays can cause you to backslide. In fact, the average person gains seven to ten pounds during the Christmas and New Year season, according to experts. The following strategies will help you keep your weight from creeping up, no matter what the holiday.

- Remember the tried-and-true rule: Don't deprive yourself; enjoy in moderation. Sweet-potato pie, cornbread stuffing, or peach cobbler calling your name? Have some, but make it a small serving. It's all about portion control. Rigidly denying yourself a little taste of holiday goodies can backfire. Why risk going overboard later? You'll really berate yourself then. Have a taste and be done with it.
- When carving up the holiday bird, go for white meat over dark (fewer calories) and always remove the skin (again, fewer calories).
- At barbecues, try not to fill up on fatty hot dogs and hamburgers. Opt for skinless chicken with a brush of tangy barbecue sauce instead.
- Here's a trick that will work for any holiday: Use a smaller plate. Your plate will look full, but you will really be eating less.
- Don't hang out by the food. Get your grub and move on. Focus less on eating and more on socializing. Remind yourself that the holidays are a time for family and friends. Use the time well.
- Remember that cocktails count too. Alcohol is loaded with empty calories. Throw back a few and you can quickly consume a meal's worth of calories without taking a single bite. Not convinced? Then consider this: 8 ounces of egg nog has about 306 calories; 12 ounces of beer has about 139 calories;

5 ounces of white wine has about 106 calories (red wine has 96); 1½ ounces of liquor (rum, bourbon, or scotch, to name a few) has about 98 calories. Keep calories in check by choosing your drinks wisely (a wine spritzer at 72 calories and a light beer at 95 calories, for instance, are better choices than their higher-calorie cousins) and not having too many of them.

- Counterbalance all the noshing with some holiday-inspired fitness. Get everyone involved. Christmastime? Go outside and have a good old-fashioned snowball fight, or take a walk and check out the neighbors' decorations. Easter? Have an Easter egg hunt in the backyard—adults only. Let the kids hide the eggs and laugh at the grown-ups running around trying to find them. Independence Day? Start your own fireworks by breaking out the hose or the sprinklers and running through the spray. Make these types of family games a new tradition. See if you and yours can think of others. The objective? To have some good physical fun. As long as you get your body moving, it counts as extra exercise.

Trigger #3—On the Job

Now here's one place where it can be very difficult to avoid triggers—the workplace. Seems as though it's always someone's birthday, or yet another coworker is getting married or having a baby. There's the company picnic, working lunches, and breakfast meetings. Whether you're toiling in a corporate environment or a service industry, the workplace is fraught with tricky situations. You can't just skip important functions. How would that look to the higher-ups? And you don't want to miss coworkers' special fêtes. You want to share in the well-wishing, not to mention get a break from your desk.

Let's not forget about the sisters who have to travel on business. Those trips offer up triggers all their own—eating airline food, ordering room service, attending meetings or conferences where the food is catered. Each situation limits your food choices, and sometimes just being away from home brings out the overindulgent tendencies in us.

Whatever your work situation, odds are you are going to have to deal with some of these on-the-job triggers from time to time. Here are a few tips to help you keep it together:

- Office parties, whether to celebrate a birthday, new baby, engagement, or big promotion, have one thing in common: cake. You probably won't have to deal with a smorgasbord of tempting entrées like you do at other parties—this is the office, after all, and work parties tend to be short and sweet, literally. Cake is the celebration food of choice on the job. Once again we have to go back to our golden rule: Moderation, not deprivation. If you really want a piece of cake (your mouth is watering just looking at it), have a sliver and savor every bite. Portion size is the key here. If you're not craving a slice of cake (maybe you recently had lunch, or you don't like pineapples, or you're not a fan of sweets, or you simply don't want any), don't feel as though you have to have a piece just because everyone else is. Politely decline and enjoy the party. Your presence is what matters most to the guest of honor, anyway.
- When it comes to important office functions—-the annual company picnic, for instance, or breakfast and lunch meetings, or conferences—make the best of the food choices available. The selection will likely be limited, so opt for the leanest cuts of meat, vegetables, green salads, fruit, pasta that's not drenched in oil, or other foods that mesh with your new eating plan. Drink plenty of water too. It will help fill you up.
- Traveling sisters may be able to make special food requests for their flights ahead of time. Call your airline and inquire; some of them will try to accommodate you. Bring along bot-

tled water and smart snacks (for example: pretzels, bananas, grapes, whole wheat crackers, chopped carrots and celery, graham crackers) in case you have to make do with what's offered and end up eating only part of the meal.

- Most hotels these days offer heart-healthy selections on their room-service menus. When ordering in, look for those items. The menu will either group heart-healthy foods into their own section, or put an asterisk or small heart next to those dishes to indicate that they are low in fat, calories, and cholesterol.

- Don't use a business trip as an excuse to cut loose. Treat it as just another day in your life. You wouldn't resume old eating habits if you were home, would you? Why do so on the road? Ask yourself that question each day you're away to help stay focused on your new, healthier lifestyle.

- Take advantage of the hotel gym. There's no reason to give up your workouts simply because you're away from home. Most major hotels have some sort of exercise facility. Or you can always swim a few laps in the pool. If all else fails, use your two feet and take a walk through the hotel and around the grounds for thirty minutes each day that you're there. You can even do calisthenics in your hotel room. You know you can come up with a way to exercise while out of town on business. Commit to it.

The Struggle Within

Whew! All of those trigger situations to deal with. It can make a sister tired just thinking about it. But once you lose weight, it's the kind of thing you *have* to think about. It's hard, we know. Reconciling yourself to the fact that these lifestyle changes are forever is no easy feat—for anyone. That's why it's so common for many sisters also to encounter a sort of "internal struggle." When you break it all down and get past the outside pressures—

the parties, the traveling, the holidays—you're left with one final truth: You have to keep the pounds off yourself. No one but you. And the smart changes you've made aren't just a quick fix; they aren't temporary. They are forever. The journey you've taken over the months or years won't end simply because you drop a certain number of pounds. The real journey will just be beginning, sister-friend. Once you trim down, you have to dig deep within yourself and find the courage and strength to maintain your fit body, your improved health, and your renewed spirit. You will have come so far, and we want you to keep going. But for some sisters, coming to terms with the infinity of the journey can be difficult. The reality is that you can't go back to your old ways and expect to keep the weight off. You have to keep moving forward. It's so easy to slip back into a detrimental way of thinking—to remember a time when you'd eat way too much and exercise far too little—and then feel a twinge of longing. *God, I can't keep this up forever,* you may think to yourself.

If you've succeeded this far and find yourself grappling with the past, take heart. You're not alone. Many other sisters out there feel the same way. They've done it. They've lost the weight and they are proud of themselves. They feel great. But they also feel like "exhaling." The truth is they—and you—already have exhaled. You've purged yourself of the destructive habits that put your health at risk. When you cracked open this book and took that first tentative step on the journey to fitness, it was your first breath—it was the first time you truly exhaled. You let your old way of thinking seep out, and allowed the information that could give you control of your life to filter in. If you could take that first step, girlfriend, you can take a million more.

Believe in yourself and let the numbers keep you inspired: Your lowering blood pressure, cholesterol count, weight, dress size. Every morning when you rise, think about how you feel physically and emotionally. Compare that to how you used to feel before you started this journey. No comparison, is it? Remind yourself of the difference each day. Most of all, don't beat yourself up if you falter. None of us can tread this path perfectly. We're going to take a misstep now and again; we're going to stumble. But we must keep on stepping. All we can do is the best we can do. As long as we put forth a good, honest effort, that's all He and anyone else will ask of us. There are no judgments here. There's only better health, a longer life, a rejuvenated spirit, and a strong, toned body. So as you turn this corner and begin your new maintenance journey, keep that in mind. Remember too, no magic pill got you to this point. Your faith, determination, and commitment did. You're taking control of your life, sister. Don't ever let go of the reins.

Sister to Sister
✕◇✕✕◇✕✕◇✕

Shirley McClendon, a fifty-year-old elementary school principal from Pontiac, Michigan
Current weight: 150 pounds
Amount lost: 50 pounds

My professional life was always great, but about nine years ago my personal life was going to pieces. I'd been married for twenty years, then it all fell apart. My marriage was deteriorating and I couldn't handle it. So I turned to food for comfort. I was eating ice cream, pie, all kinds of sweets. I tended to reach for food when I first came home from work and later at night when there was nothing to do.

I'd always been a fairly active person, but at that time I became completely inactive. I kept putting on weight and I felt miserable. I couldn't do some of the activities I'd normally do, like bowling. The weight made me so tired that I just couldn't do it anymore.

I was depressed and I didn't think anyone loved me. I

attributed it to my increasing weight. It was such a difficult time for me. But eventually I decided that my marriage was not going to be a marriage and that I had to move on. From that point, I started slowly thinking more about myself. Who I was, what I was, and how I'd changed from the person I used to be. I had to go back and refind myself.

Once I got my divorce, I took stock. I had my health. I had a home. I had three beautiful children. I had a great job. And I had the weight. I thought about all the other sisters out there who were in worse circumstances than mine, and how they had made it. I realized I had too many blessings to dwell on the past. So many times sisters put all their life into their marriage and their kids—I know I did this. We take care of ourselves last, and it should be the other way around. We need to take care of ourselves and be happy with who we are. It will make us a better person for our children. When I thought about all of that, I knew it was time for me to take care of me. It was time for me to lose the weight.

I'll admit, at that point I felt desperate. So I went to a diet center for three months, where they had me on diet pills. I did lose weight. But when I stopped going, I gained all the weight back. The pills reduced my appetite, but I didn't learn how to change my eating habits. I don't think diet pills are a healthy way to lose weight.

After that I did it on my own. Just basic things like cutting back, not having sweets (my big problem area), eating more good foods, and making sure I had breakfast in the morning. I used to skip it.

I started walking several miles each day and I did a little weight training with dumbbells.

I've kept the weight off for six years now. Once I started believing in myself and believing that I could experience good things, losing the weight became natural. There are times now when I don't feel like working out, but I keep my sneakers right by the bed so when I get up I can see them. That way I know I'll put them on and go. Once you get started, you're bound to keep going. It's all about getting out of that bed. These days when I want to snack, I don't reach for the sweets. I have pretzels instead. I love to eat ice, so I use that as another snack substitute. It keeps my mouth busy.

I also have little things I do to keep myself motivated and focused. First of all, I have this beautiful box with tulips on it. It's made to look like a present and I've had it for five years. I look at that box every day as a reminder that I'm a present to myself.

Secondly, I read *Prevention* magazine and the different fitness magazines because it's not just about weight. It's about health, and I want to stay up on that information. There are so many black women my age who are passing away from all kinds of illnesses. I believe that if we exercise, keep our weight in check, and make sure our muscles are strong—from the heart muscle all the way down—it will help us live better.

And finally, I make sure that there is a spiritual aspect to my life. Before I go to work in the morning, I read a psalm. This is something I make sure to do every day. I have a psalm for whatever mood I'm in. The twenty-third is one of my favorites.

Psalm 23
The Lord is my shepherd; I shall not want.
He maketh me to lie down in green pastures: he leadeth me
  beside the still waters.
He restoreth my soul: he leadeth me in the paths of
  righteousness for his name's sake.
Yea, though I walk through the valley of the shadow of death, I
  will fear no evil: for thou art with me; thy rod and thy staff
  they comfort me.

*Thou preparest a table before me in the presence of mine
enemies: thou anointest my head with oil; my cup runneth
over.*

*Surely goodness and mercy shall follow me all the days of my
life: and I will dwell in the house of the Lord for ever.*

APPENDIX A

How to Establish a Church-Based Weight-Loss Program

In chapter 3 we told you about the Baltimore Church High Blood Pressure Program, Lose Weight and Win, which began as a means to help Baltimore's African-American community get a handle on the health problems affecting its members, primarily cardiovascular disease and high blood pressure. The church setting was a perfect vehicle to reach the sisters of Baltimore because the church has always played such a vital role in our lives. The organizers knew a spiritual atmosphere would offer support, encouragement, and kinship to those trying to take control of their health.

Ultimately, the Baltimore church program expanded to include a weight-control component, and it proved to be an overwhelming success. Nearly every person who participated in the program lost weight. It's clear that the collective identity within the black church, which offers us strength and support, helped the folks in Baltimore successfully shed pounds. And it can do the same for you.

Today, the Baltimore program, which is now known as the Community Health Awareness and Monitoring Program (C.H.A.M.P.)

works with twenty-five churches in Baltimore, helping sisters just like you improve their health. In her work with C.H.A.M.P., project director Jeanne Charleston, R.N., has found that programs based on individual counseling and self-motivation don't work as well for black women as social, group-oriented programs. We couldn't agree more. What better place to find the fellowship, caring, and vested interest you need to reach your health- and weight-loss goals than in your house of worship?

If you would like to start a weight-loss support group or program in your church, take time to truly consider the work involved. As important a project as this is, you need to be real with yourself. It's a big undertaking. So reflect on the commitment necessary, and ask yourself honestly whether or not you are up to the challenge. You may even want to consider enlisting the help of a friend rather than going it alone. Think you can handle it? Good. We think you can too. You have committed to taking control of your own health and improving your own life, and it feels good. It makes sense that you would want to share that sense of empowerment with others, and we're so glad that you do. We sisters need to support one another in our fitness journey.

To help you get your program up and running, we brainstormed with C.H.A.M.P. project director Jeanne Charleston for insight into getting started, handling problems, and ensuring success. Let us take you through it all, step by step.

Step 1: Talk to Your Pastor

The pastor is key. Talk to him or her and explain that you are interested in starting a church-based weight-loss group and that you would like his support. Ask if the pastor would be willing to announce your planned program from the pulpit, and to discuss the importance of weight management and good health, especially for African-Americans, during the sermon. Finally, request that a notice about your new program be placed in the church bulletin. Make sure to talk to the pastor about where in the church you can hold your meetings. Have a specific room designated up-front. Your overall objective is to gain the pastor's support and help in getting the word out. Don't stop there, however. Talk it up yourself when you mingle with your fellow worshippers.

Step 2: Recruit Your Experts

You can use *Slim Down Sister* as one of your guides, but because you have to come up with an action plan that will work for a group of sisters in a structured setting, we would advise you also to seek out some tangible help from two willing-to-roll-up-their-sleeves-and-get-busy pros. First, find out if anyone in your congregation is a registered dietitian/nutritionist or a registered nurse (or L.P.N.). You will need a professional to help you map out the eating guidelines for your action plan. Also, find out if anyone in the congregation is a certified fitness trainer or has a fitness background. Again, it's important to work with an expert in developing a feasible exercise routine. Ask around. Chances are you'll find two people who can fill the bill. If you don't, someone is bound to know someone—a sister, an aunt, a friend—who has the qualifications. Or a fellow church member might work at a hospital or other health organization, and may be able to steer you to a professional who is willing to work with your group. Of course, if you can find two experts within your own congregation, all the better. The point is to start talking to people to get what you need—free of charge.

Step 3: Call a Meeting

Once the pastor has announced your plan and you have your two experts on board, call a meeting of all those interested in taking part. By now you will have heard from sisters in the congregation who want to participate in your new program. Use this initial meeting to introduce your two experts and to hammer out days, times, and length for your regular meetings. (Will you meet once a week, or twice? What times will the meetings start and end?) Allow each person to offer her input, and then come to a consensus that will work best for everyone. Be sure to decide on a time frame as well: for instance, 8 weeks, 10 weeks, 12 weeks—whatever seems right to the group. Having a concrete time frame in place gives your program structure and makes it feel "real," not like something someone just threw together. When that set number of weeks is up, simple institute a new time frame.

Step 4: Map Out the Whole Thing

Get together with your two experts well in advance of your first official group meeting, and map out a week-by-week plan for the program. What topics will be discussed each week? How will each meeting be set up? Will there be any demonstrations? Do you want to start each meeting with a few minutes of prayer? Will there be suggested readings or handouts? Will you have guest speakers on certain days? Will there be weekly weigh-ins, and if so, who will provide the scale? What goals should be set for each meeting? And so on. As you map things out with your experts, a variety of other questions will come up. Cover all the bases.

Step 5: Ready, Set, Go

Time for your first official meeting. You're bound to be excited and nervous all at the same time. Relax, girlfriend. You're getting together with sisters who love and support you. They want this to work as much as you do.

Important Points to Consider

- Even though you may have a designated spot in the church in which to hold your meetings, last-minute changes can crop up. What happens if a church function unexpectedly coincides with your group's scheduled meeting? The pastor tells you he's sorry but he needs the space that has been promised to you. What will you do then? You have to plan for these unforeseen circumstances. Figure out a backup site in advance. Some churches will be big enough to simply house your group in another room. But in a smaller church, you may have a problem. When your weight-loss program is still in the planning stages, check with a neighborhood school, community center, rotary club, or other local organization to see if they would be willing to act as your backup site. You may even want to talk to your group about designating different folks' homes as alternate sites, too (depending on the size of your group).
- Speaking of size, try to keep the number of program participants to a manageable total. If a lot of sisters in your congregation want to take part, consider breaking it up into two groups and having another person act as leader of the second group.
- On the flip side, if you only get a handful of interested sisters, think about hooking up with another church for a joint program. Speak with your pastor about the idea if you believe it's necessary.
- Try to meet at least twice a week, if possible. Don't just have a discussion group; get your bodies moving, too. Exercise is as much a vital part of weight loss as changing eating habits. You might break up one meeting this way: half discussion session, half exercise session. Then use the week's other meeting as a full exercise session. That way, your group is working out together at least twice a week. Also, encourage members to exercise on their own at least two more times

during the week. You'll have to determine how you'll fit exercise into your program during the planning phase; just remember that it needs to be an integral part of your program in order for you and the other sisters to improve your health and shed those pounds.

- Think of ways to keep your meetings interesting. Try to make them interactive whenever possible. The last thing you want is for the sisters, or yourself, to be bored. Food demonstrations are a good activity. Speak with your pastor about using the church kitchen now and then. That way you can plan to prepare low-calorie, low-fat soul-food dishes together during certain meetings. Have the nutritionist lead the discussion as you all fix the foods as a group. Then, when it's done, you can dig in.

- Invite guest speakers. This is another way to keep your meetings interesting. Check with a local hospital, university, or health club for experts who may be willing to stop by for a half-hour or so to talk with your group about a particular health or fitness topic. As with everything else, plan it in advance.

- You may want to try implementing a buddy system in which everyone has a designated partner. This is an easy, effective method of shoring up everyone's resolve and providing extra support. Say one of the sisters doesn't have a way to get to the meeting on a particular night. Maybe her husband took one car to go someplace, and her teenage daughter jumped in the other one. Well, with the buddy system, that girlfriend would have a ride. Or imagine one of the sisters is having a crisis of will—she's about ready to give up on herself and go back to old eating habits. In this scenario, she'd be able to pick up the phone and call her "buddy" for some much-needed encouragement. The buddy system is an extension of the group as a whole. It's simply a means to extend the support and sense of connection your group already provides.

- Have everyone set short- and long-term goals for them-selves. Instruct them to focus on health and behavioral goals, not weight-related ones. For example, goals may in-clude something like drinking eight glasses of water each day, or being able to walk up a flight of stairs without get-ting winded, or bringing blood pressure down.
- Use part of your meeting as a sharing session, when whom-ever wants to speak can talk about her successes or difficulties, ask questions, or pose concerns. Basically, you want to use the time to let people just talk and share their feelings with one an-other; to offer up their advice, ideas, comfort, and encourage-ment. Remember, the purpose of your program is to provide a loving, nurturing, safe place where sisters can share, learn, and, most important, take control of their health.

APPENDIX B

⌘

Slimmed-Down Soul-Food Recipes

Potato Salad

MAKES 6 SERVINGS

1 cup low-fat mayonnaise
2 teaspoons mustard
2 tablespoons vinegar
⅛ teaspoon salt
⅛ teaspoon black pepper
6 medium potatoes, cooked in jackets, peeled and cubed
1 cup celery
3 tablespoons green pepper
2 tablespoons chopped pimiento
¼ cup chopped onion

1. In a large bowl, blend mayonnaise, mustard, vinegar, salt, and pepper to make a salad dressing.
2. Add potatoes, celery, green pepper, pimiento, and onion to the salad dressing.
3. Fold together, then place into a serving bowl. Sprinkle with paprika and refrigerate.

Serving size: ½ cup; **Calories:** 144; **Fat:** 6.2 g; Calories from fat: 56; Saturated fat: 1.0 g; Cholesterol: 7.7 mg; Sodium: 152 mg; Carbohydrate: 19 g; Dietary fiber: 2 g; Sugars: 2 g; Protein: 5 g.

Macaroni and Cheese

MAKES 6 SERVINGS

2 cups elbow macaroni
2 tablespoons margarine
2 tablespoons all-purpose flour
½ teaspoon salt
2 cups skim milk
8 ounces low-fat cheddar cheese (grated)

1. Cook macaroni noodles according to package directions. Drain and place into 2-quart casserole dish.
2. Melt margarine and stir in flour and salt to make a roux, stirring constantly for approximately 3 minutes. Gradually pour in milk and stir until mixture is thick.
3. Add grated low-fat cheese (reserve ¼ cup for top of casserole) and stir until melted.
4. Mix cheese sauce with macaroni. Sprinkle top of casserole with ¼ cup of grated cheese and bake for 35 minutes at 350°F.

Serving size: ½ cup; **Calories: 277; Fat: 14 g;** Calories from fat: 126; Saturated fat: 7 g; Cholesterol: 30 mg; Sodium: 536 mg; Carbohydrate: 25 g; Dietary fiber: 0; Sugars: 3 g; Protein: 13 g.

Collard Greens

MAKES 8 SERVINGS

*1 large bunch collard greens (64 ounces cut and
washed)*
2 cups chicken broth (canned or homemade)
2 medium onions, chopped
3 whole garlic cloves, crushed
1 teaspoon red pepper flakes
1 teaspoon black pepper

1. Wash and cut greens. Mix in large stock pot with chicken
   broth, onions, garlic, red pepper flakes, and black pepper. To
   allow flavor to blend, prepare dish earlier in the day; the
   longer it blends, the better it tastes.
2. Cook at medium heat until tender (about 1 hour).

Serving size: ½ cup; **Calories:** 66; **Fat:** 1 g; Calories from fat: 11; Saturated
fat: 0 g; Cholesterol: 0 mg; Sodium: 64 mg; Carbohydrate: 14 g; Dietary
fiber: 5 g; Sugars: 3 g; Protein: 4g.

Oven-Fried Chicken

MAKES 4 SERVINGS

1 three-pound whole fryer chicken, cut into 8 serving
  pieces
1 cup skim milk
1 cup all-purpose flour
1 teaspoon thyme
1 teaspoon garlic powder
1 teaspoon onion powder
1 teaspoon parsley flakes
1 teaspoon paprika
1 teaspoon black pepper
1 teaspoon salt
⅛ teaspoon red pepper

1. Remove skin from chicken. Place in large bowl with skim milk.
2. In another large bowl, mix flour, thyme, garlic powder, onion powder, parsley flakes, paprika, black pepper, salt, and red pepper.
3. Spray a large baking pan with nonstick cooking spray and set aside.
4. Dredge chicken parts in flour mixture, making sure all pieces are well coated. Place each piece in pan. Spray top of each piece with a little cooking spray.
5. Preheat oven to 400°F. Bake for 45 minutes or until juices run clear when chicken is pierced.

Serving size: 2 pieces; **Calories:** 326; **Fat:** 9 g; Calories from fat: 81;
Saturated fat: 4 g; Cholesterol: 106 mg; Sodium: 559 mg; Carbohydrate: 20 g;
Dietary fiber: 1 g; Sugars; 2 g; Protein: 38 g.

Hush Puppies

MAKES 6 SERVINGS

2 cups yellow cornmeal
2 teaspoons baking powder
½ teaspoon salt
½ cup onions, chopped
½ cup green peppers, chopped
½ cup egg substitute
1 cup skim milk

1. Mix cornmeal, baking powder, and salt. Add chopped onions and green peppers to cornmeal mixture.
2. Combine egg substitute and milk in another bowl, then add to cornmeal mixture. Mix well, stirring until batter is stiff enough to drop from a spoon.
3. To thicken batter, add more cornmeal. To thin batter, add a little water. Drop spoonfuls of batter onto a cookie sheet that has been well coated with nonstick cooking spray. Lightly spray the tops of the hush puppies with nonstick cooking spray. Bake for 25 minutes at 400°F.

Serving size: 2; **Calories:** 172; **Fat:** 2 g; Calories from fat: 14; Saturated fat: 0 g; Cholesterol: 0 mg; Sodium: 210 mg; Carbohydrate 34 g; Dietary fiber: 5 g; Sugars: 2 g; Protein: 11 g.

Cornbread

MAKES 8 SERVINGS

1 two-ounce can jalapeño green peppers, chopped
2½ cups skim milk
2 cups egg substitute
3 cups cornmeal mix
1 cup shredded low-fat cheddar cheese
1 eight-ounce can whole-kernel corn
1 tablespoon sugar
1 teaspoon baking powder

1. Drain peppers, rinse under cold water, and chop into small pieces.
2. Blend milk and egg substitute in large bowl. Add cornmeal mix, cheese, corn, sugar, baking powder, and peppers.
3. Pour batter into a greased 13 × 9 × 2 baking pan. Bake in oven at 400°F for 35 minutes or until bread is golden brown.

Serving size 1 2 × 2-inch square; **Calories:** 217; **Fat:** 5 g; Calories from fat: 42; Saturated fat: 1.2 g; Cholesterol: 2 mg; Sodium: 479 mg; Carbohydrate: 35 g; Dietary fiber: 3.3 g; Sugars: 4 g; Protein: 9g.

Banana Pudding

MAKES 8 SERVINGS

1.5-ounce box sugar-free instant vanilla pudding
1 cup light whipped topping
3 bananas, sliced into disks
25 vanilla wafers

1. Mix pudding according to directions on the box, using skim milk when following pudding package directions.
2. Add whipped topping to the mixture and stir well.
3. Layer pudding, slices of banana, and vanilla wafers into a 2-quart glass casserole dish. Refrigerate.

Serving size: ½ cup; **Calories:** 163; **Fat:** 3 g; Calories from fat: 58; Saturated fat: 2 g; Cholesterol: 9 mg; Sodium: 238 mg; Carbohydrate: 31 g; Dietary fiber: 2 g; Sugars: 15 g; Protein: 3g.

Hoppin' John

⊗

MAKES 4 SERVINGS

1 medium onion, chopped
2 ounces smoked turkey breast, chopped
2 tablespoons olive oil
16 ounces frozen black-eyed peas
2 cups water
1 bay leaf
⅛ teaspoon black pepper
⅛ teaspoon salt

1. In a stock pot, sauté onions and smoked turkey with olive oil until onions are transparent.
2. Add black-eyed peas and water to the onion and turkey sauté.
3. Cook uncovered with bay leaf for 45 minutes at medium heat, allowing flavors to blend. Add water as necessary. When peas are done, add black pepper and salt. (To thicken: Mix 2 tablespoons all-purpose flour and 2 tablespoons water to make a paste. Add paste to peas after they have cooked 45 minutes. Simmer another 15 minutes.) Remove bay leaf. Serve over rice.

Serving size: ½ cup; **Calories:** 251; **Fat:** 8 g; Calories from fat: 79; Saturated fat: 2 g; Cholesterol: 17 mg; Sodium: 432 mg; Carbohydrate: 7 g; Dietary fiber: 2 g; Sugars: 0 g; Protein: 17 g.

Chicken and Dumplings

MAKES **6** SERVINGS

*1 three-pound whole fryer chicken, cut into serving
  pieces
¾ cup all-purpose flour
½ teaspoon salt
2½ teaspoons baking powder
1 egg, beaten
⅓ cup skim milk*

1. Cook chicken in boiling salted water in large stockpot until tender (about 30 minutes). Remove chicken. Skin and bone chicken after it has cooled. Reserve 4 cups of the broth in the pot.
2. In a bowl, combine 6 tablespoons flour with ⅓ cup chicken broth to form a paste. Add paste to the 4 cups of chicken broth, stirring until mixture is thickened.
3. To make dumplings: Combine remaining flour, salt, and baking powder in a bowl. Combine egg and milk in a separate bowl and add to the flour, stirring until ingredients are mixed well.
4. Bring chicken broth to a boil, then drop in dumpling mixture by spoonfuls. Cover and cook for 15 minutes. Add deboned chicken, simmer, and serve.

Serving size: 1 cup; **Calories:** 260; **Fat:** 10 g; Calories from fat: 88; Saturated fat: 3 g; Cholesterol: 112 mg; Sodium: 481 mg; Carbohydrate: 13 g; Dietary fiber: 0 g; Sugars: 1 g; Protein 28 g.

Gumbo

MAKES 10 SERVINGS

2 pounds okra
4 tablespoons olive oil
2 large red onions, chopped
1 medium green bell pepper, chopped
2 ribs celery, chopped
8 cups water
2 teaspoons ground thyme
2 whole bay leaves
2 teaspoons salt
1 teaspoon cayenne pepper
1 teaspoon black pepper
6 small whole blue crabs, outside shells removed
1 pound claw crabmeat
2 pounds shrimp, deveined and peeled
3½ cups rice, cooked (optional)

1. Clean okra with dry cloth to remove fuzz. Cut the ends and discard them. Cut okra into ¼-inch slices. In heavy skillet, sauté okra in 2 tablespoons of olive oil until dry, stirring occasionally. In another skillet in 2 tablespoons of olive oil, sauté red onions, green pepper, and celery until limp.

2. Combine sautéed onions, green peppers, and celery with sautéed okra in a soup pot. Add water, thyme, bay leaves, salt, cayenne pepper, and black pepper. Cook for 3 hours, stirring occasionally. Add water if necessary. Remove bay leaves.

3. Clean and split crabs. Add crabmeat, shrimp, and crabs to boiling soup and cook for 15 minutes. Serve over a mound of hot rice.

Serving size: 1 cup; **Calories:** 209; **Fat:** 7.3 g; Calories from fat: 65; Saturated fat: 1 g; Cholesterol: 139 mg; Sodium: 574 mg; Carbohydrate: 7.4 g; Dietary fiber: 0 g; Sugars: 2.2 g; Protein: 27 g.

Peach Cobbler

MAKES 8 SERVINGS

2 sixteen-ounce cans sliced peaches packed in own juice
1 cup sugar
2 teaspoons vanilla extract
1 teaspoon lemon extract
2 teaspoons cinnamon
2 teaspoons nutmeg
2 tablespoons margarine
4 tablespoons shortening
2 cups self-rising flour
1 cup fat-free buttermilk

1. To make filling: Place peaches, sugar, vanilla, lemon, cinnamon, nutmeg, and margarine in a medium saucepan and simmer for 15 minutes.

2. To make crust: In a bowl, cut shortening into flour, using two bread knives or pastry cutters, until the size of peas. Add buttermilk and mix until combined. Pour onto floured board and knead for about 3 minutes. Roll out until dough is about ⅛-inch thick.

3. Spoon about a quarter of the peaches into a 13 x 9-inch baking dish. Place a quarter of rolled dough on top of peaches, and brown in the oven at 400°F for about 5 minutes. Layer peaches on top of browned crust and place another section of rolled dough on top. Brown again for 5 minutes. Continue to layer and brown until the last crust is browned. (Optional: Serve hot with low-fat frozen yogurt.)

Serving size: ½ cup; **Calories:** 363; **Fat:** 9 g; Calories from fat: 89; Saturated fat: 2.4 g; Cholesterol: 1.2 mg; Sodium: 451 mg; Carbohydrate: 66 g; Dietary fiber: 0 g; Sugars: 26 g; Protein: 5 g.

Catfish Stew

MAKES **6** SERVINGS

2 garlic cloves, crushed
½ teaspoon oregano
¼ teaspoon dry mustard
dash of cayenne pepper
4 pounds catfish, filleted
2 tablespoons olive oil
1 can tomato soup
1 cup water
¼ cup catsup
1 tablespoon Worcestershire sauce
½ cup onion, chopped

1. In a small bowl, mix garlic, oregano, mustard, and cayenne pepper. Sprinkle mixture on fish.
2. Brown catfish fillets on both sides in olive oil. Remove from pan.
3. Add tomato soup, water, catsup, Worcestershire sauce, and onion to pan. Bring to a boil.
4. Add catfish and simmer for 30 minutes or until fish separates. Do not stir mixture. Lift catfish to prevent sticking or scorching. Serve with hot brown rice.

Serving size: 1 cup; **Calories:** 424; **Fat:** 10 g; Calories from fat: 161; Saturated fat: 4 g; Cholesterol: 175 mg; Sodium: 536 mg; Carbohydrate: 7 g; Dietary fiber: 0 g; Sugars: 1.3 g; Protein: 55 g.

Southern Chopped Barbecue

MAKES 10 SERVINGS

5 pounds fresh Boston butt pork roast
1 teaspoon parsley
½ teaspoon dill weed
1 tablespoon garlic powder
1 tablespoon onion powder
2 teaspoons black pepper
Your favorite barbecue sauce

1. Rinse pork roast and pat dry.
2. In a small bowl, mix parsley, dill weed, garlic powder, onion powder, and black pepper. Rub mixture onto pork roast.
3. Place pork roast on a rack in a baking pan (fat will drip into the pan). Bake at 350°F for 1 hour. Do not add any sauce or salt to meat prior to cooking.
4. Remove bones and chip the pork as you desire. After chipping, add barbecue sauce to taste and serve.

Serving size: 3 oz; **Calories:** 375; **Fat:** 15 g; Calories from fat: 125; Saturated fat: 5 g; **Cholesterol:** 133 mg; Sodium: 473 mg; Carbohydrate: 5 g; Dietary fiber: 0 g; Sugars: 0 g; Protein: 33 g.

Shrimp Fried Rice

MAKES **4** SERVINGS

1 pound medium shrimp
1 tablespoon olive oil
½ cup chopped green onions
½ cup chopped onions
½ cup green bell pepper
1 egg, beaten
3 cups cooked rice
3 tablespoons light soy sauce
1 teaspoon powdered ginger
½ teaspoon ground black pepper

1. Peel and devein shrimp, then rinse well.
2. In a dutch oven, heat olive oil over medium heat. Add shrimp and sauté until pink. Remove and set aside.
3. In the same pan, sauté all onions and bell pepper until tender (approximately 3 to 4 minutes). Remove vegetables from pan and set aside.
4. Scramble the egg, then add cooked rice, vegetables, shrimp, soy sauce, ginger, and black pepper. Stir until mixed well. Continue stirring until mixture is heated through.

Serving size: 1 cup; **Calories:** 326; **Fat:** 7 g; Calories from fat: 61; Saturated fat: 1.3 g; Cholesterol: 218 mg; Sodium: 520 mg; Carbohydrates: 36 g; Dietary fiber: 0; Protein: 28 g.

Grandma's Smothered Chicken

MAKES 4 SERVINGS

1 three-pound whole chicken
1 teaspoon salt
½ teaspoon black pepper
1 cup flour
2 tablespoons olive oil
½ cup celery, chopped
1 cup onions, chopped
3 garlic cloves
2 cups chicken broth
1 teaspoon thyme
½ teaspoon sage

1. Cut chicken into serving sizes. Rinse pieces and pat dry with paper towels. Season with salt and pepper.
2. Pour flour into a paper bag. Add chicken pieces to bag and shake to dust chicken with flour. Remove chicken from bag and shake off excess flour.
3. Heat a large skillet until hot, then add olive oil and chicken. Brown chicken on both sides. (Cook only until chicken is browned, not well cooked.) Remove chicken from pan and set aside.
4. Add celery, onions, and garlic to pan and sauté. After sautéing the vegetables, place chicken in pan and add the chicken broth, thyme, and sage. Cook until chicken is tender and juices run clear (approximately 20 to 25 minutes).

Serving size: ¼ chicken; **Calories:** 428; **Fat:** 16 g; Calories from fat: 145; Saturated fat: 3.4 g; Cholesterol: 112 mg; Sodium: 109 g; Carbohydrates: 7.2 g; Dietary fiber: 2 g; Protein: 40 g.

Curry Chicken

MAKES 6 SERVINGS

1 three-pound fryer, cut into pieces
2 tablespoons olive oil
½ cup onion, chopped
2 garlic cloves, minced
2 teaspoons paprika
3 teaspoons curry powder
1 teaspoon cumin
1 teaspoon salt
¼ teaspoon black pepper
⅓ teaspoon ground cinnamon
½ cup water
2 teaspoons cornstarch
1 apple, peeled and chopped

1. Add olive oil and chicken pieces to a hot skillet and brown chicken on both sides.
2. Remove chicken from skillet and set aside. Add onions and garlic to the skillet and sauté until onions are translucent.
3. Stir in paprika, curry powder, cumin, salt, black pepper, and cinnamon. Add the browned chicken. Pour in water and simmer until chicken is tender (about 30 minutes).
4. Thicken gravy with cornstarch and 4 tablespoons of water. When chicken is tender, add apples. Serve over rice.

Serving size: ¼ chicken; **Calories:** 193; **Fat:** 8 g; Calories from fat: 71; Saturated fat: 2 g; Cholesterol: 79 mg; Sodium: 468 mg; Carbohydrates: 5 g; Dietary fiber: 1 g; Protein: 25 g.

Pork Tenderloin with Apples

MAKES 6 SERVINGS

½ pound pork tenderloin
1 teaspoon garlic powder
1 teaspoon fennel seeds
1 teaspoon thyme
1 teaspoon salt
1 teaspoon ground ginger
½ teaspoon black pepper
¼ cup red wine
2 cups apples
½ cup sugar
¼ cup brown sugar
1 teaspoon cinnamon
2 teaspoons nutmeg
1 teaspoon vanilla

1. Wash tenderloin and pat dry.
2. In a small bowl, combine garlic powder, fennel seeds, thyme, salt, ginger, and black pepper to make a dry rub. Rub tenderloin thoroughly with seasoning mixture.
3. Place tenderloin in an oven-ready pan and add wine. Bake at 350°F until well cooked (about 35 minutes).
4. In a separate pan, brown apples. Add sugar, brown sugar, cinnamon, nutmeg, and vanilla. Cook until apples are soft.
5. Serve with apples spooned over tenderloin.

Serving size: 3 oz; **Calories:** 322; **Fat:** 17 g; Calories from fat: 154; Saturated fat: 6 g; Cholesterol: 110 mg; Sodium: 480 g; Carbohydrates: 14 g; Dietary fiber: 1 g; Protein: 29 g.

Meatloaf with Soul

MAKES 6 SERVINGS

½ pound extra-lean ground beef
1 pound ground turkey
1 teaspoon Worcestershire sauce
1 tablespoon prepared mustard
2 teaspoons salt
1 teaspoon black pepper
1 medium onion, grated
¼ cup green bell pepper, chopped
¾ cup oatmeal
1 egg, whole
½ cup evaporated skim milk
½ cup catsup

1. Combine ground beef, turkey, Worcestershire sauce, mustard, salt, black pepper, onion, and bell pepper in a large bowl. Mix thoroughly.
2. Add oatmeal, egg, and milk. Mix thoroughly, then shape into a loaf. (Wetting your hands with water will keep ground beef from sticking to your hands.)
3. Bake at 350°F for 1 hour. During the final 10 minutes, brush meatloaf with catsup.

Serving size: 3 oz; **Calories:** 341; **Fat:** 17 g; Calories from fat: 158; Saturated fat: 6.3 g; Cholesterol; 139 mg; Sodium: 559 mg; Carbohydrates: 10 g; Dietary fiber: 1 g; Protein: 34 g.

Corn Pudding

MAKES 4 SERVINGS

2 cups frozen whole-kernel corn
1 cup 1-percent milk
2 eggs, whole
½ teaspoon salt
¼ teaspoon black pepper
1 tablespoon margarine
2 tablespoons sugar
2 tablespoons flour
¼ teaspoon nutmeg

1. Lightly grease a baking dish and place corn in dish.
2. In a small bowl, combine milk, eggs, salt, black pepper, margarine, sugar, and flour.
3. Pour mixture over corn kernels and sprinkle with nutmeg. Set baking dish in large pan. Pour enough water into pan to reach one fourth of the way up the sides of the baking dish. Place pan in 325°F oven and bake for 45 minutes. When a knife comes out clean, the corn pudding is done. Let stand for 3 minutes, then serve.

Serving size: ½ cup; **Calories:** 200; **Fat:** 7 g; Calories from fat: 60; Saturated fat: 2 g; Cholesterol: 112 mg; Sodium: 525 mg; Carbohydrates: 30 g; Dietary fiber: 2.1 g; Protein: 7.8 g.

Baked Sweet Potatoes

MAKES 4 SERVINGS

4 sweet potatoes, in jackets
2 teaspoons olive oil
¼ cup brown sugar

1. Rinse sweet potatoes and dry with paper towels.
2. Rub potatoes with oil and place on an ungreased baking sheet.
3. Bake at 400°F until potatoes are soft (about 1 hour). Remove potatoes from oven. Cut open and add brown sugar for a sweet Southern taste.

Serving size: 1 potato; **Calories:** 250; **Fat:** 2 g; Calories from fat: 25; Saturated fat: 0 g; Cholesterol: 0 mg; Sodium: 27 mg; Carbohydrates: 13 g; Dietary fiber: 2.1 g; Protein: 3 g.

Seasoned Grilled Fish

MAKES 4 SERVINGS

4 white-fish fillets (cod, flounder, snapper, etc.)
2 garlic cloves, minced
1 teaspoon parsley flakes
½ teaspoon salt
1 teaspoon tarragon
1 teaspoon thyme
½ teaspoon black pepper
¼ cup lime juice from fresh limes
2 tablespoons light soy sauce
1 teaspoon mustard
⅓ cup canola oil

1. Wash and dry fish fillets.
2. In a small bowl, combine garlic, parsley flakes, salt, tarragon, thyme, and black pepper. Rub the dry seasoning mixture onto fish.
3. In another bowl, combine lime juice, soy sauce, mustard, and 1 tablespoon of the canola oil. Place fish fillets in a shallow pan and drizzle the lime-juice mixture over the fillets.
4. Place pan on grill (gas grill or charcoal grill can be used with water-soaked wood chips), cover, and cook 5 to 6 minutes. Turn fish over and cook an additional 5 to 6 minutes. Check for doneness: When fish is opaque, it's done. Serve immediately.

Serving size: 4 oz; **Calories:** 310; **Fat:** 7 g; Calories from fat: 136; Saturated fat: 1 g; Cholesterol: 97 mg; Sodium: 525 mg; Carbohydrates: 0; Dietary fiber: 0; Protein: 40 g.

Smothered Cabbage

MAKES 6 SERVINGS

1 large head of cabbage
¼ cup olive oil
½ cup onion, chopped
1 green pepper, quartered
1 teaspoon sugar
1 teaspoon salt
1 teaspoon caraway seeds
½ teaspoon black pepper
¼ cup water

1. Cut cabbage in half, remove core, wash, then shred coarsely.
2. Heat oil in large skillet; sauté the onions and green pepper for about 10 minutes.
3. Add cabbage, sugar, salt, caraway seeds, and black pepper, and continue to sauté for a few more minutes.
4. Add water, reduce heat, and cover pan. Cook until cabbage is tender (about 15 minutes).

Serving size: 1 cup; **Calories:** 119; **Fat:** 9 g; Calories from fat: 83; Saturated fat: 1 g; Cholesterol: 0 mg; Sodium: 417 mg; Carbohydrates: 8 g; Dietary fiber: 4 g; Protein: 2 g.

Smoked Turkey Collard Greens

MAKES 4 SERVINGS

4 pounds collard greens
4 cups chicken stock
¼ pound smoked turkey breast
1 cup onions, chopped
3 garlic cloves, minced
1 jalapeño pepper, whole
½ teaspoon black pepper

1. Clean and wash greens thoroughly. Stack and roll leaves, then cut crosswise into strips.
2. Place chicken broth in a large pot. Add smoked turkey, onions, and garlic. Boil for 10 minutes.
3. Add greens, jalapeño pepper, and black pepper. Reduce heat and cook until tender (approximately 1 hour).

Serving size: 1 cup; **Calories:** 118; **Fat:** 2 g; Calories from fat: 15; Saturated Fat: 0; Cholesterol: 16 mg; Sodium: 479 mg; Carbohydrates: 16 g; Dietary fiber: 2 gs. Protein: 13 g.

Aunt Sarah's Buttermilk Peach Pie

MAKES 8 SERVINGS

1 unbaked 9-inch pie crust
1 teaspoon vanilla extract
1 teaspoon lemon extract
1 cup sugar
3 tablespoons flour
1 cup low-fat buttermilk
2 eggs
3 tablespoons margarine
4 peach halves

1. Prepare pie crust by pricking it and baking for 5 minutes. Remove from oven and cool.
2. In large bowl, combine vanilla and lemon extracts, sugar, flour, and buttermilk. Mix well.
3. In a small bowl, beat the eggs. Melt margarine and add to the beaten eggs.
4. Add egg and margarine mixture to buttermilk mixture and mix well.
5. Place peaches in pie shell with the cut sides facing up. Pour buttermilk mixture into pie shell. Bake at 425°F for 15 minutes, then reduce heat to 350 degrees and bake for another 30 minutes. When knife comes out clean, pie is done. Cool and serve.

Serving size: 1 slice; **Calories:** 199; **Fat:** 5 g; Calories from fat: 51; Saturated fat: 1 g; Cholesterol: 49 mg; Sodium: 81 mg; Carbohydrates: 35 g; Dietary fiber: 0 g; Protein: 3 g.

Sweet Potato Pie

MAKES 8 SERVINGS

2 large sweet potatoes, in jackets
4 tablespoons butter or margarine
2 teaspoons lemon juice
2 eggs
1½ cups sugar
12-ounce can skim evaporated milk
1 teaspoon vanilla
2 teaspoons cinnamon
2 teaspoons nutmeg
1 unbaked 9-inch pie crust

1. Place sweet potatoes in a pot and boil until potatoes are soft (approximately 20 minutes).
2. Once potatoes are done, put them aside. When potatoes are warm, peel them and place in a bowl. Add butter and lemon juice and mash together.
3. To mashed potato mixture add eggs, sugar, milk, vanilla, cinnamon, and nutmeg. Blend until creamy.
4. Pour filling into pie shell and bake in a 350°F degree oven for 1 hour or until knife comes out clean and pie is lightly brown on top. Cool and serve.

Serving size: 1 slice; **Calories:** 360; **Fat:** 8 g; Calories from fat: 77; Saturated fat: 2 g; Cholesterol: 47 mg; Sodium: 192 mg; Carbohydrates: 64 g; Dietary fiber: 2 g; Protein: 7 g.

Bread Pudding

MAKES 8 SERVINGS

8 slices whole wheat bread
1 cup evaporated skim milk
2 teaspoons vanilla extract
2 eggs
1 cup sugar
2 teaspoons butter extract
16-ounce can peach slices

1. Tear bread slices into pieces.
2. Add milk, vanilla extract, and eggs to the bread pieces and mix well.
3. Add sugar, butter extract, and peaches to the bread mixture. Mix well.
4. Place bread mixture into a well-greased pan. Bake at 350°F for 1 hour or until bread pudding is browned. Cool and serve.

Serving size: 1 cup; **Calories:** 387; **Fat:** 4 g; Calories from fat: 32; Saturated fat: 0; Cholesterol: 93 mg; Sodium: 274 mg; Carbohydrates: 85 g; Dietary fiber: 6 g; Protein: 8 g.

Low-Fat Sour Cream Pound Cake

MAKES **24** SLICES

3 cups sugar
¾ cup margarine, soft
1⅓ cup egg substitute
1½ cup low-fat sour cream
1 teaspoon baking soda
4½ cups sifted cake flour
¼ teaspoon salt
1 tablespoon vanilla extract
1 tablespoon butter extract
2 teaspoons lemon extract

1. Blend sugar, and margarine at medium speed until smooth.
2. Gradually add egg substitute. Beat well.
3. In a separate bowl, combine sour cream and baking soda. Stir well and set aside.
4. In another bowl, combine flour and salt.
5. With mixer running at low speed, begin alternately adding sour-cream mixture and flour mixture to cream mixture. Begin with the sour-cream mixture and end with the flour.
6. Stir in vanilla, butter, and lemon extracts.
7. Spoon batter into a tube pan that has been sprayed with nonstick spray. Bake for 1 hour at 325°F. Cool and remove from pan.

To make a glaze: Combine powdered sugar with the juice of 1 fresh lemon. Mix well and pour over cooled cake.

Serving size: 1 slice; **Calories:** 250; **Fat:** 7.7 g; Calories from fat: 53; Cholesterol: 6 g; Sodium: 152 mg; Carbohydrate: 42 g; Protein: 3.5 g.

Black-Eyed Peas with Smoked Turkey

MAKES 6 SERVINGS

1 pound dried black-eyed peas
½ pound smoked turkey
1 onion, chopped
1 teaspoon sage
½ teaspoon salt
½ cup green pepper, chopped
½ teaspoon black pepper
1 bay leaf
1 garlic clove, minced

1. Rinse black-eyed peas thoroughly. Place smoked turkey, onions, peas, and water to cover in a pot and boil until beans are tender (about 3 hours). Add additional water if necessary.
2. Add sage, salt, green peppers, black pepper, bay leaf, and garlic. Cook for 30 more minutes. Serve over rice.

Serving size: 1 cup; **Calories:** 147; **Fat:** 2 g; Calories from fat: 14; Saturated Fat: 0 g; Cholesterol: 16 mg; Sodium: 520 mg; Carbohydrates: 19 g; Dietary fiber: 2 g; Protein: 14 g.

Stewed Okra, Tomatoes, and Corn

MAKES 6 SERVINGS

1 pound fresh okra
2 large tomatoes
1 onion, chopped
½ green pepper, chopped
½ teaspoon black pepper
½ teaspoon paprika
1 teaspoon sugar
1 cup water
16-ounce package frozen corn

1. Discard stem and ends from okra and slice.
2. Peel and slice tomatoes.
3. In a skillet sprayed with nonstick cooking spray, sauté okra until browned.
4. Add onion, tomatoes, green pepper, black pepper, paprika, sugar, and water. Bring to a boil.
5. Add corn, reduce heat, and simmer for 15 minutes.

Serving size: ½ cup; **Calories:** 117; **Fat:** 0; Calories from fat: 7; Saturated Fat: 0 g; Cholesterol: 0 mg; Sodium: 13 mg; Carbohydrates: 26 g; Dietary fiber: 4 g; Protein: 5 g.

Mashed Potatoes with a Hint of Garlic

MAKES 4 SERVINGS

4 large potatoes
½ cup skim milk
3 garlic cloves, chopped
½ teaspoon black pepper
½ teaspoon salt

1. Peel potatoes, cut into pieces, and cook in boiling water for 20 minutes or until tender. Drain and return to pot.
2. Mash potatoes, adding milk, garlic, black pepper, and salt as you mash. Mix until smooth (or desired texture). Serve hot.

Serving size: ½ cup; **Calories:** 127; **Fat:** 0; Saturated fat: 0 g; Cholesterol: 0 mg; Sodium: 315 mg; Carbohydrates: 28 g; Dietary fiber: 2 g; Protein: 3 g.

Pinto Beans

MAKES **4** SERVINGS

½ pound smoked turkey breast
2 cups water
2 pounds dried pinto beans
1 large onion
1 garlic clove, minced
2 teaspoons celery seeds
1 teaspoon black pepper
⅛ teaspoon salt

1. In a large pot, boil the turkey in 2 cups of water for 15 minutes.
2. Add pinto beans, onion, garlic, celery seeds, and black pepper. (Do not add salt yet. Adding salt during the cooking process makes the beans hard.) Cook until tender (ap mately 1 hour).
3. When beans are tender, add salt. Try serving

Serving size: 1 cup; **Calories:** 251; **Fat:** 2.2 g; Calories f
fat: 0 g; Cholesterol: 18 mg; Sodium: 429 mg; Carbohyd
fiber: 6 g; Protein: 20 g.

Baked Pork Chops

MAKES 4 SERVINGS

1 cup wine vinegar
1 tablespoon olive oil
1 teaspoon ginger
1 teaspoon prepared mustard
1 teaspoon pepper
1 teaspoon oregano
1 teaspoon basil
1 teaspoon parsley flakes
1 teaspoon cumin
⅛ teaspoon salt
1 teaspoon sugar
4 pork chops, lean
1 onion, sliced

1. To make marinade: In a large bowl, combine vinegar, olive oil, ginger, mustard, pepper, oregano, basil, parsley flakes, cumin, salt, and sugar.
2. Place pork chops in marinade and refrigerate for 2 hours. Drain marinade and place chops in a baking dish. Bake at 350°F for 30 to 45 minutes, adding sliced onions during the last 10 minutes of cooking.

Serving size: 1 pork chop; **Calories:** 301; **Fat:** 15 g; Calories from fat: 118; Saturated fat: 5 g; Cholesterol: 66 mg; Sodium: 292 mg; Dietary fiber: 0 g; Protein: 19 g.

Green Beans with Onions

MAKES **6** SERVINGS

2 tablespoons corn-oil margarine
2 pounds fresh green beans
1 large onion, sliced
1 cup water
1 teaspoon salt
1 teaspoon pepper
1 teaspoon dill weed

1. In a skillet, melt margarine and then sauté green beans and onions for 3 to 4 minutes.
2. Add water and cover. Cook for 20 minutes or to the doneness you desire. Add salt, pepper, and dill weed, and serve.

Serving size: ½ cup; **Calories:** 81; **Fat:** 4 g; Calories from fat: 35 g; Saturated fat: 0 g; Cholesterol: 0 mg; Sodium: 246 mg; Carbohydrates: 11 g; Dietary fiber: 3.2 g; Protein: 2 g.

Acknowledgments

My thanks goes out to many people who have helped me along the way. To Curtis, my husband and friend: Thank you for being the rock of support in my life. Thanks also to the loves of my life Candace and Curtis (CJ) for giving me the time I needed to work on the book. Thanks to my biggest cheerleading squad, my sisters Rojean, Althea, Willa, Julia, Sakina. Your support and words of encouragement are priceless. To my in-laws Zelma Weaver, Isabelle Christain, and Eddie James Weaver (my second dad)—thank you, thank you, thank you. To my neighbor, Theresa Daniels, thanks for being the substitute mom for the kids when I had trips or meetings. I love you girl. To my Pastor, the Reverend Walter R. Prince Jr., and his wife, Dianne Prince, your prayers went up and the blessings came down. Thanks for believing in me and giving me the ability to see that God does great things through having faith and believing that God gives us all the things we really need. To the members of Mt. Pleasant Missionary Baptist Church, Orlando, Florida, your support and kind words are deeply appreciated. I'm proud to belong to a church that practices heart-healthy deeds of services in the church and community. To my many friends and relatives, Theresa, Charles, Maleika, Laverne, Michael, Alex, Rogelle, Mike, Alex Jr., Tamieka, Shadale, Dan, Danielle, Brittany, Joel, Austin, Connor, Zachary, Everette, Everette III, Jerome, Jeffrey, Tony, Robert, Valerie, Thelma, Mary B., Mary R., Lillian, and many more relatives and friends of the Williams–Weaver clan. You guys have been there for me when I needed help or just when I needed someone to listen to my ideas. I love you all. To Fab, the most special person that came into my life over ten years ago. I would have never imagined that we would have made as terrific a team as this. You are my sister in many ways. Together we have made many dreams come true. To my personal photographer, Sherman Sheffield, God has blessed you with many talents; have faith and believe and you will go many places. To Angela, a miracle happened when we met you. Your talents and skills are unique, and God has given you the ability to put it all on paper. You are the best! To Linda Konner, thanks for representing the both of us; your help means a lot to us. To the many people that I have touched or helped along the way, your thoughts were instrumental in the development of this book. Thank you all.

—R.W.

This book would not have been possible without the love and encouragement of many people. To my husband, Charlie A. Gaines—thanks for all your love and devotion. You are my biggest cheerleader and I love you very much. To my son, Tramaine—you are the son every mother hopes for. Thanks for being a wonderful son. To my daughter, Devona—God is preparing you for bigger and better things. To my brother, John L. Demps Jr., and sisters Eunice Demps and Jeanette Demps Hudson—I love you guys, thanks for all the support. To my lifelong friends Deborah Jean Mitchell, Vavescia Johnson, Felecia Williams, Shirley Bouie-Lee, and Almeda Jefferson—we are not getting older but better. Thank you for listening to me. To my cousin Cynthia Holmes—you are like a sister to me. Thanks for being you and believing in me. To my mother-in-law, Mary Alice Gaines—thanks for your prayers and wisdom. I love you for everything you do in my life. Special thanks to all my aunts and uncles on the Demps, Sirmans, and Holmes side of my family. You are my rock of support. Finally, thanks to Roniece Weaver for being the wind beneath my wings and giving me the opportunity to use my creative thinking and for listening to all my crazy ideas. I love you like a sister; may God continue to bless and keep you and your family. To Angela—thanks for giving me the opportunity to write this book with you. You are a wonderful person and I know with God's help you will go far.

—F.G.

All of my love to my mother and father, Shirley T. Ebron and Peter Ebron. Thank you for always believing in me. A heartfelt thank you to a wonderful agent, Linda Konner, for her wisdom, guidance, support, and friendship. Many thanks to Cheryl Solimini for opening the door. A great big thank you (big up!) to Michael Lewis for his crazy sense of humor and his encouragement. You kept me sane. Thanks to Yvette Chavis (hey girl), Sandy Prysby, Valerie Reid, Deborah Brockett, Janene Moore Patterson, and Judy Watson-Remy for putting me in touch with the "sisters." Thank you to Mara Hoskin-Thomas for her help and expertise. Many, many thanks to Roniece and Fabiola, two of the sweetest, most down-to-earth sisters I've ever met. You made this a pleasure from start to finish. God Bless.

—A.E.

Recipe Index

General Index